i

The Whole Tooth

Answers to the questions you always wanted to ask your dentist

Martin Thomas Nweeia,
D.D.S., F.A.C.D., F.I.C.D., F.A.D.I., F.P.F.A., F.A.G.D.

Fellow of the American College of Dentists
Fellow of the International College of Dentists
Fellow of the Academy of Dentistry International
Fellow of the Pierre Fauchard Academy
Fellow of the Academy of General Dentistry

Illustrations by Kevin Hand

Made possible in part by a grant from
the Hawaii Dental Service Foundation

CASTLE BOOKS

This edition published in 2005 by
Castle Books ®
A division of Book Sales, Inc.
114 Northfield Avenue
Edison, NJ 08837

Originally published by
Randall Morita Design
866 Iwilei Road, Suite 206
Honolulu, HI 96817

Published by arrangement with
Dr. Martin Nweeia, D.D.S.
The Whole Tooth ©
P.O. Box 35
Sharon, CT 06069

This book is intended to be a reference only and not a substitute for a dentist's
professional opinion regarding your dental needs. All readers should
consult with a dentist before undertaking any form of self-treatment.
Likewise, they should consult their dentist before beginning or discontinuing
any medication described in this book.

Any brand name listed in this publication does not represent an endorsement
of the product, nor does the omission of a brand name signify any criticism.

ISBN-13: 978-0-7858-1964-6
ISBN-10: 0-7858-1964-9

Printed in the United States of America

For Kristen and Katya

About the Author

Dr. Martin Nweeia has won several writing awards including the International College of Dentists Golden Pen Award and the Editorial Award of Excellence from the Academy of General Dentistry. He has received the Community Service Award from the Academy for his work with Hawaii's homeless and continues assisting the less fortunate as Dental Director of the Volunteers in Medicine Clinic, Berkshires.

Recognized for his dental research, Dr. Nweeia has led dental field expeditions to the Colombian Amazon, Ulithi Atoll in Micronesia and most recently a series of expeditions to the Canadian Arctic to study the elusive narwhal, known for its unicorn-like spiraled tusk. He was a Joseph Silber Fellow from the American Cancer Society, a grant recipient from the National Science Foundation and the National Endowment for the Arts and a National Fellow of the Explorers Club, World Center for Exploration.

Dr. Nweeia graduated from Trinity College in Hartford and received his doctorate from Case School of Dental Medicine. His postdoctoral training was completed in Sweden. Dr. Martin Nweeia practiced dentistry for 11 years in Honolulu serving on the State Board of Trustees and as Editor of the Hawaii Dental Journal. He currently practices in Sharon, CT and serves on the Board of Governors and as Editor of the CT State Dental Journal. He is clinical instructor of the Advanced Dental Rotation at the Harvard School of Dental Medicine.

About the Artist

Kevin Hand continues as graphic designer in the second edition of The Whole Tooth. He began his career in 1982 working at several newspapers in Florida including Florida Today in Melbourne. Kevin continued as graphic designer for The Honolulu Star-Bulletin in Honolulu, Hawaii, and the Chicago Tribune in Chicago, Illinois. Kevin has won several awards including Society of News Design awards for informational graphics in 1991 (Arizona Memorial), 1997 (Inside Chicago's Symphony Hall), and 1998 (Nagano Olympics: Snowboarding). He has won international recognition for graphics in the breaking news category with Malofiej design competition in Pamplona, Spain for his work in 2000 (Elian Gonzales raid), 2001 (Long Island American air crash), 2002 (Inside the Church of the Nativity). In 1998 Kevin was involved in a Chicago local news project that ultimately won the Pulitzer Prize for staff writer Blair Kamen. Kevin now produces informational graphics and illustration for Newsweek Magazine in New York City. His work can also be seen in respected publications such as Popular Science and Men's Journal magazines. Kevin is married and living in Brooklyn, New York.

Introduction

We are all curious about our health. Yet our desire to learn is often frustrated, confused or lost when we search for answers to our most common questions. How many times have you gone to the doctor's office feeling awkward about asking a question? Perhaps you felt your question wasn't intelligent enough, or you were worried about taking too much of the doctor's time. Some physicians and dentists communicate well and encourage questions, but many do not. The flow of questions about health issues then finds other channels.

People are starving for health information in the public media. During my years as a columnist for Gannett and as a correspondent for CBS, the health sections were the most read and watched. Why? The language was simple and the illustrations and graphics were friendly and informative. Television news stories were told by ordinary people going through medical procedures. They helped us to feel at ease confronting our own feelings about going through such experiences.

References and guide books are also gaining popularity among people looking for answers to their questions. But often these books are overwhelming—long, heavy and formal. I enjoy reading about health and still find myself shying away from reading guide books. Although some health guides have relaxed their format a bit, many still have too much small-typed text and medical jargon.

People who do not enjoy the typical health reference now have the option of getting their answers from the internet. The web-based health sites often have information that is well presented with colorful and engaging graphics. Many of these sites, however, do not represent mainstream thought and the viewer can be further confused. Other sites from government health agencies and medical and dental libraries suffer from the same condition as the guide books that are published by them. They are often text only or have limited graphics. The writing is also stilted and formal.

I started recognizing these communication barriers and wanted to address them directly in this dental guidebook. I wanted to create a source that would encourage people to find answers and share experiences that would stimulate and nurture further interest. I began writing and corresponding for news agencies and saw the public hunger for health news. Later, I started to examine the format of the consumer reference and realized that in an effort to stay dignified and well respected, medical writers pushed people away. I went a step further and thought, why can't a dental guide be fun and interesting at the same time?

I have always been excited by my profession and am passionate about letting others know. The Whole Tooth is my answer to the shortcomings of health guidebooks and other sources of information. The title and illustrations are deliberately fun and friendly. Yet the information is well researched and reviewed by distinguished medical and dental experts. There is a piece in this book for everyone: the inquisitive consumer, the fearful patient, the person who has never visited the dentist, children of all ages, the disabled and people from all racial backgrounds. I hope this reference book is comfortable on your coffee table and gives you and your family an enjoyable way to explore the world of oral health.

Table of Contents:

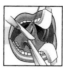

Chapter 15: Bite and Jaw Joint Problems 153

Chapter 16: Partial and Full Dentures 167

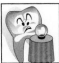

Anatomy Of A Tooth

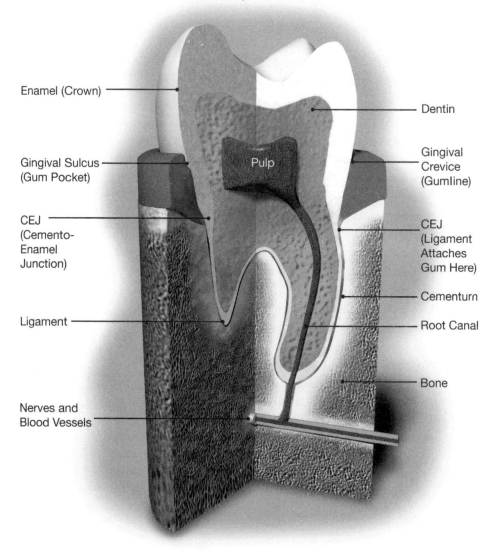

Enamel (Crown)

Dentin

Gingival Sulcus (Gum Pocket)

Gingival Crevice (Gumline)

Pulp

CEJ (Cemento-Enamel Junction)

CEJ (Ligament Attaches Gum Here)

Cementurn

Ligament

Root Canal

Bone

Nerves and Blood Vessels

Primary Teeth

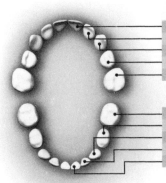

Upper Teeth	Erupt	Shed
Central incisor	8-12 months	6-7 years
Lateral incisor	9-13 months	7-8 years
Canine (cuspid)	16-22 months	10-12 years
First molar	13-19 months	9-11 years
Second molar	25-33 months	10-12 years

Lower Teeth	Erupt	Shed
Second molar	23-31 months	10-12 years
First molar	14-18 months	9-11 years
Canine (cuspid)	17-23 months	9-12 years
Lateral incisor	10-16 months	7-8 years
Central incisor	6-10 months	6-7 years

Permanent Teeth

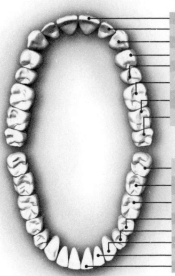

Upper Teeth	Erupt
Central incisor	7-8 years
Lateral incisor	8-9 years
Canine (cuspid)	11-12 years
First premolar (first bicuspid)	10-11 years
Second premolar (second bicuspid)	10-12 years
First molar	6-7 years
Second molar	12-13 years
Third molar (wisdom tooth)	17-21 years

Lower Teeth	Erupt
Third molar (wisdom tooth)	17-21 years
Second molar	11-13 years
First molar	6-7 years
Second premolar (second bicuspid)	11-12 years
First premolar (first bicuspid)	10-12 years
Canine (cuspid)	9-10 years
Lateral incisor	7-8 years
Central incisor	6-7 years

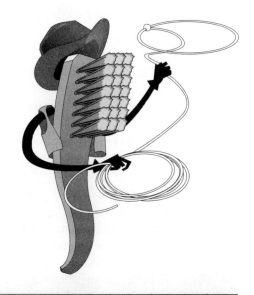

Chapter 1

Oral Hygiene

Right technique helps brush problems away

What is the proper way to brush your teeth? I've read so many explanations that seem to conflict with each other.
Also, how many times should you brush a day?

Dr. Charles C. Bass, formerly a medical school dean, described the "right way" to brush back in 1943. That technique still remains the standard among dental professionals.

Four instructional steps simplify the "Bass Technique." First, to clean the outside surfaces of teeth, hold the brush at a 45-degree angle, with the bristles contacting the area where the gums meet the tooth. Then using small circular strokes with light pressure, slowly move toward the biting edge of the tooth. The inside surfaces of the lower teeth and the outside surfaces of the upper-back teeth are the most difficult areas to clean.

To remove plaque from the inside surfaces of your front teeth, hold the brush vertically and move back and forth against the tooth. You should maintain the 45-degree angle of bristles to the tooth surface. Finally, to clean the biting surfaces of your teeth, place the toothbrush bristles directly on the surface while making small circular strokes.

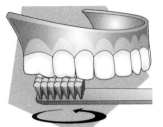

BITING SURFACE BRUSHING

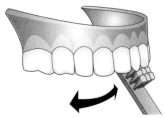

INSIDE SURFACE BRUSHING

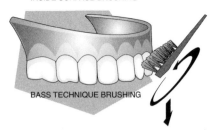

BASS TECHNIQUE BRUSHING

Other brushing techniques may be adapted for special problems like gum recession. In such cases, your dentist or hygienist will instruct you so that brushing does not further aggravate a condition. On an average, you should brush two to three times a day, depending on the health of your gums and teeth and your ability to properly clean them. Brushing correctly is more important than the number of times you brush. Your hygienist or dentist can point out areas that need additional attention.

Two frequent problems are applying too much pressure when brushing and abrading the gums with back-and-forth brush movements. With proper guidance, good brushing habits can help ensure a lifetime of dental health.

Teeth's best allies are toothbrush and floss

With all the dental devices and mouth rinses available, is there some perfect combination that I should be using to clean my teeth?

The best combination of products to clean your teeth include a toothbrush and floss and, as options, a mouthwash and a rubber-tipped device. The first two are absolute necessities. A mouthwash also can be used after flossing and brushing but should not be considered a substitute for either of these procedures. A rubber-tipped instrument or wooden stick called a Stimudent helps massage and exercise the gums. In general, good technique for brushing and flossing is better than following claims of advertisers and new products.

Look for the ADA seal on brushes, toothpastes and mouth rinses as a guide for approved products that are backed and tested by research. Although fluoride was considered the only beneficial ingredient in toothpaste, some new compounds may prove to be advantageous. Tartar control toothpastes can reduce the amount of calculus (calcified plaque) by as much as 30 percent.

When laying on paste, "a little dab'll do ya. . ."

What's the best toothpaste?
How much should you put on your toothbrush?

No toothpaste is the best. Just choose one with fluoride. Newer toothpaste products contain ingredients that supposedly cut down on plaque, whiten teeth and include agents that destroy cavity-causing bacteria. The real effectiveness of these products will not be known until long-term studies have been completed.

Many gum specialists agree that the health advantages of toothpastes alone are minimal. Avoid toothpastes that advertise cleaner, whiter teeth; often, there is little support to those claims.

A narrow one-inch ribbon of toothpaste on the toothbrush is sufficient. Advertisements during the past 20 years have shown increasing amounts of toothpaste on the toothbrush. Current ads show a full ribbon, with an additional swirl back onto itself. But in this case, more is not necessarily better. Many researchers agree that an amount less than a one-inch ribbon is adequate.

Toothpastes address more preventive needs

I have a hard time keeping my teeth clean. Do these
tartar control toothpastes and bacteria fighting rinses really work?

Yes, but they will not replace the job of brushing and flossing. The ingredients in these new products help prevent the formation of deposits on your teeth. Tartar control toothpastes, for example, contain additives that reduce the calcium and phosphate deposits which collect on your teeth. Once this hardened mineral, tartar, attaches to the teeth, it can only be removed by your dentist or hygienist.

Plaque, unlike tartar, can be removed with home care and is the target of good oral hygiene practice. Since this layer of bacteria is a cause of tooth decay and gum disease, efforts have concentrated on removing plaque with the introduction of new ingredients.

Preventing gingivitis is another claim of these products. Gingivitis, an early gum disease, is an inflammation or body reaction to the bacteria found in plaque and tartar. Since this disease is reversible, efforts to remove plaque and tartar may also prevent gingivitis and reduce the chance of more serious gum disease like periodontitis. With so many products to choose from, you should ask your dentist for recommendations.

Special toothpastes ease gumline pain

My teeth are sensitive along the gumline when I brush them.
What can I do to stop the pain?

If your discomfort occurs only when you brush and is along the gumline, you may have an exposed area of dentin. Dentin is a tooth layer underneath the outer layer of tooth enamel. Enamel is very thin by the gumline and can be worn away by abrasion from hard-bristled toothbrushes or aggressive brushing.

How can you ease the sensitivity? The easiest way is with the help of toothpastes that treat sensitive teeth. These work in a couple of ways. Those with potassium compounds work by blocking pain impulses from the nerves in your teeth. The pain is there, but your brain doesn't get the message.

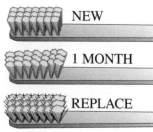

Should your pain persist or if you notice any irregular areas along the gumline of your teeth, such as grooves or notches, see your dentist. He or she may want to place some fluoride on the area to prevent any future decay. If the worn area on the tooth surface is large enough, your dentist may want to bond the area with a filling material.

If the area becomes more sensitive or begins to react to cold or hot foods, you should contact your dentist promptly.

Worn toothbrushes may irritate gums

I've been using my toothbrush for about a year now and would like to know how I can tell when it is time to get a new one?

NEW

1 MONTH

REPLACE

The answer to your question varies with each individual. As an average, you should change your toothbrush every three to four months. When you notice fraying or bending of the bristles, even if before the three- or four-month intervals, you should purchase a new brush promptly. Continued use of a brush with worn bristles may irritate the gums.

Soft bristle toothbrushes are recommended and you should ask your dentist or hygienist to suggest a brand name. Electric toothbrushes are also useful particularly for these people with limited hand dexterity.

As a general rule, you should be brushing at least twice daily for three to five minutes. If you find your toothbrush wears out more often, this may be a warning sign of an incorrect brushing technique. You may be brushing too vigorously. Toothbrush bristles usually are not damaging to tooth enamel but can be a factor in gum recession. Patients who brush vigorously often have early signs of gum recession and may even have a notch created near the gumline. This is caused by the abrasion of the brush against the gums or the root of the tooth. Such abrasion may cause tooth sensitivity and accelerate gum disease.

Bad brushing habits can irritate the gums

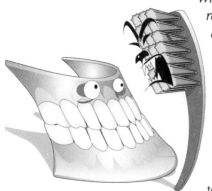

Why are the gums around my canine teeth receding, even though I brush three times a day? I'm more confused because my dentist and hygienist tell me there is hardly any plaque on my teeth when I come in for my six-month checkup.

Gum recession is most often caused by a buildup of plaque and bacteria around the teeth. But the source of your problem is more likely an irritation of your gums during improper tooth brushing.

Gingival recession can occur when heavy pressure is applied during tooth brushing or when the bristles are moved back and forth across the gums. When signs of irritation are observed, you should modify your style of tooth brushing. Hold the brush at a 45-degree angle at the gumline, then apply light pressure, moving the brush away from the teeth in a slight circular motion. This avoids continued irritation. Your hygienist or dentist can demonstrate the various ways of brushing and may ask that you demonstrate your brushing technique during your appointment to insure a proper technique.

Proper care of brush limits spread of germs

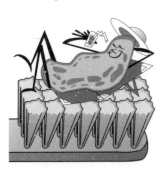

I've seen advertisements for toothbrush cleaners that keep bacteria from forming on a toothbrush. Are these valuable? Is it possible to get a disease from a toothbrush?

Although the benefits of tooth brushing far outweigh the risks, there are problems that improper brushing may cause. If a toothbrush is not properly rinsed after cleaning, it may become a future source of disease. Flu, trench mouth, herpes and colds are but a few of the afflictions that a toothbrush may spread. Toothbrushes are commonly exposed in the most germ-infected area of the home, the bathroom.

Following these tips will limit the spread of bacteria and viruses by a toothbrush:

• Choose clear or transparent toothbrushes over opaque ones that retain more bacteria.
• The fewer the bristles on a brush, the less likely bacteria will be trapped.
• Rinse your brush thoroughly after every use, and store in a dry place. Keeping the brush near a source of ultraviolet light also helps to kill bacteria.
• Change your toothbrush every few months. If you get sick, throw away your old toothbrush when you are well again.

Ideally a toothbrush should be stored outside the bathroom. If kept dry and in a plastic container, you will limit the chances of spreading germs.

Flossing is a snap if you have a right gap

I'm always trapping food between my last two lower teeth.
Even when I floss, the strand frays and sometimes breaks.
What causes this?
How can it be corrected?

Trapping food between teeth indicates a wide or rough surface between the teeth. Normally, the contact area between the teeth is tight so that the floss snaps through. If the floss easily passes between the teeth without any resistance, it can be a food trapping area. Likewise, rough tooth surfaces of either your natural tooth or filling material may also catch food. If there is a wide space, a filling may be needed to bring the contact surfaces of the teeth closer together.

Rough surfaces between teeth can sometimes be smoothed or contoured by your dentist. However, often a new filling is needed which can be made with a new smooth contacting surface. Halitosis, fraying of floss and bleeding gums all may indicate problems between teeth. More diligent hygiene is needed to keep these areas clean until the problem is corrected. If left untreated, further complications such as gum and tooth infection will result. Simple procedures often correct these problems and restore the area to a healthy state.

Flossing can pinpoint problems with fillings

While I was flossing my teeth, one of my fillings came out.
My dentist tells me to floss, but if my fillings come out,
should I avoid flossing certain areas?

If a filling comes out during flossing, you've done yourself a preventive service. Fillings are designed to withstand vertical stresses from flossing. If they come out, usually it is because of decay underneath. In some cases, though, a tiny portion of the filling may chip off, creating an area where decay can set in.

Your dentist cannot always predict these trouble areas because x-rays often do not show smaller areas of decay beneath fillings. If decay does show up on an x-ray, your dentist will remove the filling and replace it after taking the decay out. This type of decay, referred to as "recurrent decay," commonly occurs from lack of cleaning around the margins of a filling.

A recurring problem with decay around or beneath old fillings may be a warning to improve oral hygiene. Flossing removes plaque from between the teeth. If your floss frays or breaks easily, you may need to change the type of floss you use. In some cases continued difficulty when flossing may suggest an early stage of recurrent decay. As a filling or tooth breaks down, the surface edges become rough and inconsistent. The floss that grabs onto this edge may fray or work to remove a weakened filling.

Frayed edges on fillings can snag while flossing.
If the filling comes out, it may mean something more
serious like recurring decay underneath is present.

Specialized tools help make flossing easier

I'm 74 years old and have difficulty flossing my teeth.
Is there anything that makes flossing easier?
Can you recommend another way to keep my teeth clean?

You may want to purchase a floss holder, a U- or V-shaped plastic handle which tightly holds a small strand of the floss. You can floss this way with one hand. Using a different type of floss may also help. Everything from thin unwaxed floss to waxed dental tape is designed for various spaces between your teeth. One type of floss is embedded with fluoride to deposit this protective mineral between teeth.

If an area is not clean after repeated flossing attempts, you may need other cleaning tools. Floss threaders, for example, are plastic loops which help thread the floss underneath bridges and teeth that are splinted or fused together for support. Proxibrushes are miniature versions of a toothbrush. These help clean awkward areas that may be impossible to clean. Dental toothpicks also are useful, but you must be careful not to poke or irritate the gums.

If continued efforts are still not working, ask your dentist for some guidance. Rather than explain your problems, demonstrate to your dentist the difficulty you have. Often correcting a technique can solve the dilemma. Likewise, have your dentist demonstrate any new device or method of oral hygiene. Despite efforts to communicate the value of flossing, recent studies concluded that nine out of ten Americans still do not floss once a day as recommended.

Water Piks are useful but brushing is better

I want to buy my husband a Water Pik for Christmas. He has a hard time brushing sometimes, and I thought this would help him clean his teeth. Do you recommend Water Piks?

DYNAMIC DUO

Water Piks or other oral irrigating devices are useful for loosening food debris around the teeth or partial dentures and bridges. The forced water spray helps clean orthodontic braces that trap food. Water Piks do not remove plaque and tartar and so should never be considered a substitute for brushing. It's like cleaning a dirty car. If water is sprayed on the car, large debris will come off, but a sponge or brush is needed to remove the dirt. You may also want to consider an electric or ultrasonic toothbrush. These enable a more thorough cleaning for people who have little manual dexterity or simply prefer an electric method of doing a manual chore. If your husband has a hard time brushing, one of these may be a preferred option.

Should you decide to buy an oral irrigating device, there are two types. One has a self-contained pump. The other attaches directly to your faucet. Ask your dentist to recommend a pressure setting and frequency of use. There are also rinses that can be used instead of water in the self-contained machines. Again, ask your dentist for recommendations.

Dental implants need special care at home

*I have dental implants in my lower jaw now, and I've been finding it
difficult to clean around the implants after eating certain foods, like beef.
Should I be using special instruments?*

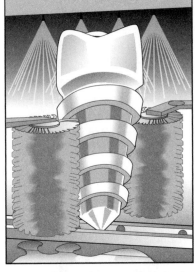

Your dentist or hygienist can suggest special cleaning instruments or floss and can order them if they aren't available at your pharmacy. Small interproximal toothbrushes can help clean hard-to-reach spaces between implants. Antimicrobial mouth rinses also may help.

Be sure any device you plan to use meets with the approval of your dentist and never use metal instruments, which can damage the soft titanium implant material. Even during regular cleanings, hygienists and dentists use plastic instruments that will not irritate or damage the gums or implants.

Proper home care is the best defense against infection, which may loosen the support around the implants. Like the roots of natural teeth, implants can become infected and may even be lost if not properly cared for. Because gum and bone diseases in the mouth are usually not painful, regular dental checkups are necessary.

Sugarless gum helps fight cavities, but. . .

*Our son showed us an article that said
sugarless gum helps fight tooth decay.
Is this true?*

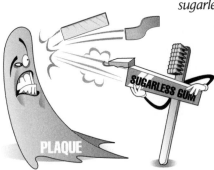

Several studies suggest that sugarless gum may help prevent tooth decay. Bacteria in the mouth feed on sweets and starches and produce acids which cause cavities. Eating foods with sugar can cause damage to the teeth in minutes; starches don't damage teeth for several hours.

Researchers found that if sugarless gum is chewed after eating sugar or starch, the amount of harmful acids produced would decrease. Gum also creates more saliva, which acts as the body's natural defense against cavity-causing bacteria. There are some disadvantages to sugarless gum. Certain sugar substitutes may cause stomach distress. Constant gum chewing can also place undue stress on certain dental restorations and appliances. Be sure to consult with your dentist.

Heredity plays a part in cavity resistance

My daughter brushes her teeth regularly, yet she has as many cavities as my son, who eats a lot of junk food. Why?

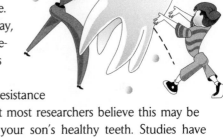

Although a healthy diet is important to reducing chances of tooth decay, other factors may play a bigger role. Inherited resistance of teeth to decay, good oral hygiene and fluoride supplements all can help reduce a child's chances of developing cavities.

Genetic traits associated with the resistance to tooth decay is difficult to prove. But most researchers believe this may be part of the answer and may explain your son's healthy teeth. Studies have shown, for example, that certain ethnic groups have thicker tooth enamel, which would help guard against penetration by tooth-attacking bacteria.

Oral hygiene usually explains differences between individual rates of tooth decay. For that reason, brushing and flossing are stressed as a defense against tooth decay. No amount of inherited resistance or good eating habits will prevent destruction of the teeth if bacteria are allowed to remain undisturbed on tooth surfaces.

Numerous studies indicate that fluoride supplements make the outer enamel surface of teeth more resistant to decay. By binding to the teeth during development, fluoride helps prevent bacteria from starting cavities.

Maximizing all your defenses gives you an advantage against tooth decay. Your son can further limit cavities by developing good eating habits. Have your daughter continue her good dental care because becoming lazy will likely result in further decay.

Chlorhexidine is an effective mouthwash against bad breath

What is the best mouthwash to use? The store shelves are filled with brand names that have all sorts of claims on their labels. Are these claims accurate and how much do they matter in choosing which one to use?

The number of mouthwashes on the store shelves has increased threefold in the past ten years. Claims vary from freshening breath to fighting plaque and gingivitis to preventing cavities.

Consumer Reports tested 15 mouthwashes to evaluate how effective they are for fresh breath. Results were so varied that none proved consistently better than another.

For reducing plaque and gingivitis, mouthwashes containing chlorhexidine were thought to be the most effective, according to the American Dental Association's Council on Dental Therapeutics. Peridex, available by prescription only, is an example of such a rinse. Studies indicate that these rinses may be effective against volatile sulfur compounds, anaerobic bacteria associated with halitosis or bad breath. Other rinses which commonly contain phenolic compounds also reduce plaque. However, these may not be as effective as chlorhexidine rinses.

Sodium fluoride in mouthwash seems to be the most effective agent in preventing cavities. Because of the positive research results from studies on both fluoride-containing toothpastes and mouthwashes, the ADA now recommends that children over the age of six rinse and brush daily with these products.

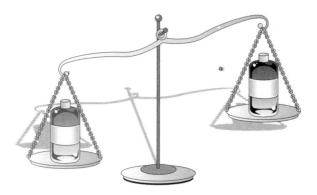

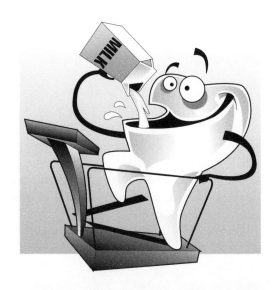

Chapter 2

Diet and
Dental Nutrition

Eating right is a factor in preventing decay

How much of the saying, "You are what you eat,"
applies to people who get a lot of cavities?

That depends on how a "good diet" is defined,
say the experts. It may surprise you, but
malnourished people in many poor countries have
lower rates of tooth decay than well-nourished populations
in the United States. A study in a famine area of India, for
example, found 75 percent of the 12-year-old children free
of cavities. In contrast, only one percent of children were
found to be free of cavities in Rochester, NY Teeth
apparently do not break down from dietary
deficiencies as do other parts of the body.

When people in underdeveloped countries adopt the
diets of developed countries, they do get more cavities, probably because they
begin consuming more sugar. Dental experts have focused on reducing sugar
and carbohydrate intake to cut tooth decay.

Other dietary nutrients have been associated with oral health. A lack of
vitamin C has been associated with periodontal or gum disease. Insufficient iron
can result in a fungal infection. And inadequate amounts of fluoride and
calcium may also increase your cavity risk.

Calcium is important to keeping teeth healthy

Can the calcium in dairy products help make your teeth stronger?
I've heard that calcium is good for stronger teeth and bones.

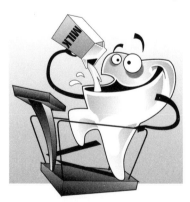

There's mixed truth to that statement.
Your bones probably benefit more from dietary
calcium than your teeth. Calcium supplements
are beneficial in preventing osteoporosis and
maintaining bone mass and strength throughout your life.

Your dentist may recommend additional
calcium supplements during or after surgical operations such as tooth extractions and gum surgery
to aid the body in its bone healing. Dairy products
rich in calcium can be important in this role.

The balance of calcium in teeth is much less understood. The statement that more calcium makes stronger teeth is a myth. Still, calcium plays an important role. For example, "remineralization" is a process by which tooth decay is reversed by the reincorporation of calcium and phosphate to the weakened area. Remineralization is dependent on calcium in the saliva. Your dentist commonly places a layer of calcium solution at the base of deep cavities before placing a new filling to help the tooth repair itself and adapt.

Certain cheeses like Swiss, Monterey Jack and aged cheddar may have decay-fighting components. Rich in calcium, cheeses also contain fatty acids, phosphates and proteins, all believed to be a part of this cavity-fighting property. Although the importance of calcium should not be underestimated, there have been no studies proving that increased dietary intake will make your teeth less susceptible to tooth decay.

Artificial sweeteners help keep you smiling

Do artificial sweeteners reduce your chances of getting cavities?

Chances of getting cavities are greatly reduced when you substitute artificial sweeteners for sugar in your diet. The bacteria that cause cavities feed on sugar, then produce acids which weaken the outer layer of the tooth and eventually cause a hole or cavity.

Most sugar substitutes are not like these basic sugars that cavity producing bacteria can use. Are there risks associated with substitutes? Little evidence exists to challenge the safety of artificial sweeteners now in use. Studies so far have not turned up dangers strong enough to overcome consumer demand. Cyclamate, for example, has a controversial past and was at one time banned in the United States for its possible link to cancer. But evidence was weak enough, and consumer and corporate demand powerful enough, that Cyclamate returned to the marketplace. Until many of the newer artificial sweeteners have been used for several years, it's difficult to comment on the possible long-term risks.

Vegetarian diet plays a role in oral well-being

*We'd like your help to resolve a debate
at our house. Do vegetarians have less
tooth decay than meat eaters?*

Recent studies indicate that vegetarians average a significantly lower number of cavities when compared with those who eat meat. However, the absence of meat in a diet may not be the single important factor explaining the reported differences. Vegetarians who consume a lot of soda pop, sweets and junk food may be just as prone to cavities.

A study of 1,200 children in South India reveals differences in diet as they may relate to tooth decay. Seven and a half percent of the vegetarians had developed cavities compared to 42 percent of the non-vegetarians.

Vegetables in the diet have been associated with many other health factors in the gums and teeth. Among more recent findings is the relationship between vitamin A commonly found in many vegetables and fruits and a reduced risk of oral cancer. Oral cancer patients treated at the University of Arizona had a marked reduction of the cancer.

Many studies showing the relationship between diet and oral health reinforce the value of the well-balanced diet.

Diet plays limited roles in gum maintenance

*My husband was told by our dentist that
he had bad gum and bone disease in his jaws.
He doesn't eat right, and I've told him
that besides brushing his teeth, he needs
to have a good diet. Isn't that true?*

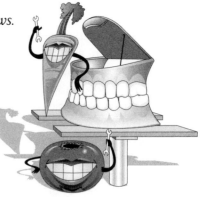

Yes, but more studies are needed to give a clear picture of the relationship between diet, and gum and jaw bone health. The two nutrients that play an especially important role in the mouth are vitamin C, or ascorbic acid and calcium.

Vitamin C has been the most widely studied. When adequate amounts of vitamin C are stored in the gums, they are better able to resist destructive bacteria, and gum cells are better able to produce collagen which helps maintain this resistance.

Calcium supplements can help prevent gum and bone loss, a problem especially serious for denture wearers. Reports indicate that the bone ridges that support dentures can weaken more rapidly when calcium is lacking. Dairy products such as milk, cheese and yogurt are good sources of calcium.

Other vitamins and minerals have produced varied results. Protein supplements are found to increase gum health, whereas carbohydrates and fats have no effect. Only under the guidance of a dentist, physician or nutrition specialist should you develop a regimen for taking vitamin supplements.

And keep in mind that a balanced diet only helps your body resist infection. Oral hygiene and heredity also play important roles in bone loss and gum recession.

Tooth decay: A juicy topic for fruit lovers

I thought fruit was good for you, but a friend disagrees saying it can cause cavities. Who's right?

You're both right. Fresh fruit is considered to be an important dietary component. But recent studies revealed that cavity rates increase among avid fruit consumers.

This is believed to be caused by the acid content of fruits, which set up an environment for tooth decay. Many fruits also contain residues which attach to the teeth and must be properly cleaned or brushed away.

However, fruit has the opposite effect on your gums, increasing their health. Researchers say that fibers in apples or stone cells in pears may cleanse gum tissue. Also, important vitamins and minerals found in many fruits may be an added health benefit for your gums.

Those who avidly drink fruit juices may share some of the same benefits and consequences, although they may not have been studied to the same degree as fruit consumers.

Over a long period, juice may erode the outer enamel of front teeth. This is caused by the constant flow of juice containing natural mild acids. The erosion usually starts by the gumline and can lead to tooth sensitivity or decay. People who consume a couple of glasses of juice each day should not be concerned.

Tannin in tea and foods help fight decay
Do tea drinkers really have less tooth decay?

Several studies show that tea has anti-decay properties. Tannins are the reason. A recent University of California report found that they prevent bacteria from attaching to the tooth surface, which prohibits up to 85 percent of decay-causing bacteria from feeding on the tooth.

Researchers discovered the unique properties of tannin while studying the chewing sticks Nigerian tribes used to clean their teeth. Because they had little tooth decay, researchers expected to find a fluoride like component in the sticks. Instead, they discovered the benefits of tannins, which also may be found in apples, beer and chocolate.

Studies prove grandma right about cardamom
*My Swedish grandmother tells me that cardamom spice
in her bread is good for the gums and teeth. Any of this true?*

Cardamom is a spice that has been used by the peoples of the Middle East for centuries. It was chewed like tobacco and used in everything from mouth rinses to soaps and shampoos. Other cultures more recently incorporated the spice in cooking. Cardamom seed is used quite often in Scandinavian sweet breads and pastries.

Recent investigations at the University of California at Berkeley reveal that cardamom has ingredients that are effective against bacteria that cause tooth decay. The researchers specialize in spices that double as folk remedies for common medical conditions. The oil in the cardamom seed has also been tested and found effective against bacteria associated with scalp conditions and acne.

Chewing cardamom has long been associated with masking bad breath. But this recent study shows new proof of bacteria-fighting properties that may uphold such claims as your grandmother's.

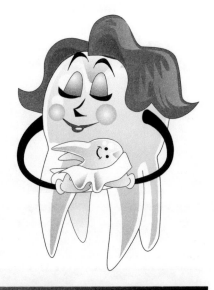

Chapter 3

Infant and Child Care
Pediatric Dentistry

Gradual introduction to a dentist is best

Does a four-year-old need to see a dentist if her teeth are not bothering her? She is very healthy and is never sick at school. We want to take good care of her teeth.

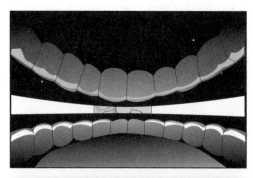
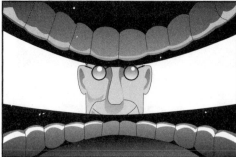
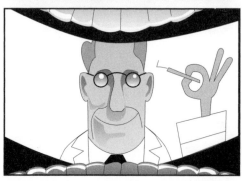

Start thinking about regular visits to the dentist when your child is two years old. Often no treatment is needed at this age, but such visits allow the child to become acquainted with the dentist and the dental environment. The child then forms a positive, trusting relationship with the dentist and will feel relaxed in the dentist chair.

Many nervous, fist-clenching, forehead-sweating adult patients would be far more comfortable had they been introduced to dentistry at a much younger age. As children, they were first brought in to see the dentist when they had a toothache. The pain and unfamiliar surroundings were traumatic enough for them to associate subsequent visits with fear and discomfort. Early and regular childhood visits allow your dentist to take a more preventive approach to dental problems, minimizing the need for emergency or more painful procedures.

The first appointment may include a combination of a short visual exam, teeth cleaning and x-rays. Prescription fluoride supplements may also be given to help prevent decay. Both general dentists and pediatric dentists (specializing in children) can meet the needs of your child.

Low levels of fluoride are carried in breast milk

*Does breast milk contain fluoride? I am now breast-feeding
our three-month-old son. Should he be getting any fluoride
supplements during this period?*

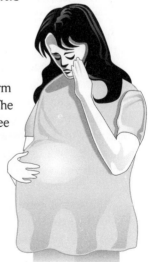

Human breast milk can provide low amounts of fluoride. Fluoridated water consumption and dietary sources
of the mother are some of the factors that determine how
much fluoride is contained in breast milk. If you live in a
non-fluoridated community, your breast milk may not
contain sufficient quantities of fluoride to help protect
your child's teeth. In such cases, fluoride drops that can be
added to your child's drinking water or juice, may be prescribed by your dentist or pediatrician.

As a general rule, while breast-feeding, use prescribed fluoride only if
you live in a non-fluoridated community. After you discontinue breast-
feeding, you should provide your child with additional sources of fluoride.
Likewise, too much fluoride should be avoided. Check with your dentist
on a fluoride supplement program that will give your child the necessary
recommended amounts.

Mom's dental visit is usually safe for fetus

*I'm pregnant and am not working now.
Would this be a good time to get some
dental work done and is it safe?*

Although most procedures are safe to perform
during pregnancy, certain times are preferable. The
fourth to sixth month are the safest, while the first three
months are riskier since the developing fetus is especially vulnerable to any changes in its environment.

X-rays and local anesthetics used during
pregnancy are usually safe. Depending on the
urgency of your dental needs, your dentist will
select an appropriate time for treatment. With
standard lead aprons, there is virtually no risk
of radiation exposure to the fetus.

All anesthetics carry a warning for pregnant women. Although generally regarded as safe, anesthetics still may affect the developing embryo. Pharmaceutical companies are conservative in their warning descriptions for the Physicians Desk Reference, the standard resource text for physicians and dentists.

During the final months, it may be uncomfortable to sit in the dental chair for a prolonged period of time. But failing to visit the dentist for the entire length of your pregnancy may place you at risk for oral infections. You should visit your dentist early in the pregnancy to map out a course of treatment that will reduce unexpected problems. Your dentist will balance your health needs with those of the fetus.

Babies' dental health is affected before birth

I'm two months pregnant and concerned about eating
the proper foods so my baby will have good teeth and bones.
Should I be taking supplements like calcium?
I've heard that if the baby isn't getting enough calcium
that it will get extra amounts from the mother's teeth and bones.
Is that true?

Not entirely. While it's true that your baby needs calcium for proper development, the sources are the mother's diet and bones, but not the mother's teeth. Likewise, the old wives' tale that a tooth is lost for every pregnancy has no truth to it. If you experience more decay when you are pregnant, it may be because you are neglecting your own oral hygiene. Frequent snacking may also be a source of an increase in cavities.

Teeth begin to form by the sixth week of gestation, and at birth many of the baby teeth are completely developed. Your concern about eating the proper foods is wise. Vitamins and minerals such as phosphorous and calcium are required by your unborn child. When you eat a balanced diet, these nutrients help both you and the baby. Try to follow these guidelines:

- Brush and floss daily to maintain your own oral health.
- Eat a balanced diet.
- Stay away from sweets and starches because they promote further decay.
- Continue regular visits to your dentist.

Childhood sickness leaves a mark on teeth

Our daughter has a permanent brownish line across two of her front teeth. What causes this? What can be done to correct it?

The line on your child's teeth may be a permanent record of an illness she has had as an infant. Often, disease or injury can affect developing teeth. The illness is thought to interfere with or upset the formation of enamel, which covers the teeth.

Just as rings on a tree define periods of growth, so do layers of enamel on teeth. Depending where the line is located, and on which teeth, your dentist can tell about when the disease or injury

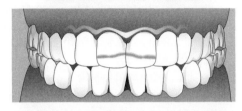

Marks of an Illness

An illness in infancy or childhood can affect developing teeth with discoloration. The illness is thought to interfere with the early formation of tooth enamel.

occurred. The closer the line is to the edge of the teeth, the earlier the injury occurred. The thickness of the line tells how long the illness lasted.

Medical problems such as hearing loss, nutritional deficiencies and respiratory problems all have been correlated with tooth lines. Since most teeth develop during the last few months of pregnancy until two years of age, diseases during this period are usually seen as brown lines. Although the brown line is more noticeable, yellow and chalky white lines mark a less severe illness.

This discoloration runs deep into the enamel, so polishing or scraping is ineffective. To cover these areas, your dentist can perform simple bonding procedures using tooth-colored material. These lines are not any more prone to decay.

One-on-one rapport with children is needed

I recently took our three-year-old daughter to the dentist, and the receptionist asked that she go in by herself. Why would they prefer that I do not accompany my child?

Your dentist is not making an unusual request. Many dentists prefer treating children alone. Making this clear before you enter the office helps avoid uncomfortable feelings with the office staff at the time of the visit.

When a parent is present during treatment, children tend to be more demonstrative than when alone. Procedures a parent may interpret as stressful for the child are often very routine. In many cases, children show no sign of fear when parents are not present.

In an attempt to comfort or hold the child, parents can make it difficult for the dentist to work. The situation becomes more complicated when children attempt to create conflict between the dentist and parent to avoid what they may perceive as a painful experience. However, some children are genuinely fearful and may benefit from a parent's presence. Your dentist can make this determination.

It's understandable that parents would want to be with their child, but children should be allowed to form their own patient-dentist relationship, an important element in lifelong dental care.

Moms with cavities can infect children

My dentist, after examining both me and my 18-month-old daughter, suggested that I take good care of my teeth because bacteria from my cavities could be transmitted to her. I've never heard of this before, is it true?

Your dentist is correct in recognizing the possible effects of caries, the disease associated with cavities, as a transmissible disease. The bacteria found at sites of tooth decay and gum disease is capable of being spread not only to other parts of your own mouth, but to another mouth. These bacteria are infections similar to those in other parts of the body. This is why certain gum and bone disorders may be treated with the aid of antibiotics.

Recent studies from the Alabama Institute of Dental Research and the University of Goteborg in Sweden have shown transmission of tooth bacteria from parents to children through genetic comparisons, similar to matching bar codes on grocery labels.

Research is unclear as to how caries is transmitted, but chances are good it is carried in saliva. As such, caries would be transmitted when a parent kissed a child. You would be wise to take your dentist's advice. Proper care on your part will benefit your teeth as well as limit the transmission of bacteria from your mouth to your child's.

Baby-bottle decay is a major concern for preschoolers

*When we pick up our child at preschool, I see so many children
with metal caps on their front teeth. Why?*

The most likely reason is baby-bottle decay. This
occurs when babies are allowed to drink sweetened
liquids from bottles for hours each day. Continuous
flow of sugar-containing liquid like soda or juice
causes a characteristic pattern of tooth decay
which can be so extensive that children need the
equivalent of root canal treatment to prevent
further destruction of the baby teeth or adult
teeth. After the root canal or pulpectomy, a
stainless steel cap or crown is placed over
the tooth. In some cases, the tooth must
be removed.

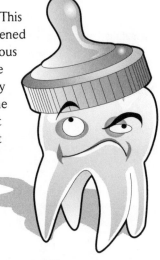

The American Academy of Pediatric
Dentistry now advises parents to have their
children checked by a dentist by age one, rather
than age two as was previously recommended.
By two, significant decay may already be present.
In addition, parents should wean their children
off baby bottles by age one.

*Baby bottles can
be detrimental to a child's
dental health if filled with
sweetened liquids.*

Babies lose sleep over teething discomfort

*My baby had a fever for several days from teething.
I think one of her teeth is not coming out fast enough.
Is there anything I can do?
Should I see a dentist when this happens?*

An old wives' tale saying that teething causes a high fever is not true.
However, babies often lose sleep while teething and don't eat and drink as
much, making them more susceptible to infection. Although your dentist can
provide you with information and treatment for the mouth, the source of
infection in these cases is often from other parts of the body. Your baby's
physician should check any sources of ongoing fever.

Teeth Evolution

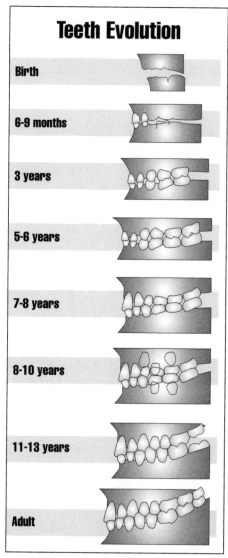

Birth

6-9 months

3 years

5-6 years

7-8 years

8-10 years

11-13 years

Adult

Teething usually begins around three to four months of age and comes and goes with varying frequency over a two-year period. Early signs of teething include drooling and dribbling. Babies also may spit up saliva or vomit more frequently. Some infants may have loose stools from swallowing excessive amounts of saliva. Other babies develop coughs during sleep as a result of saliva dripping back into the throat. Such irritation and continual saliva flow can make a child restless during the day and while sleeping.

To relieve this discomfort, let your baby chew on a hard roll, teething ring or pretzel. Cooling these devices before use soothes the affected area. Rubbing your finger across the gums also helps. Special anesthetic solutions rubbed on the gums may also provide relief. Should your baby awaken from a cough while teething, raise the head portion of the crib.

Many parents and grandparents watch for the eruption of teeth in their baby. Although there are some general guides for expecting certain teeth to appear, there is seldom a cor-relation between tooth eruption and normal infant development.

Listed here is a general guide of when you can expect certain baby teeth to appear:

- Two lower-front teeth (incisors), at six to seven months
- Four upper front teeth, at seven to 12 months
- Two additional front teeth and four molar teeth, two upper and two lower, at 14 to 16 months
- Four canine or eye teeth at 18 to 21 months
- Four second molars, at 24 to 30 months

Preventive care halts damage to sweet tooth

I am careful with the meals I prepare for my children.
Which foods, besides candies and sweets are bad for your teeth?

There are many dietary contributors to tooth decay. Almost any food can potentially damage your teeth. Eating habits are therefore as important as the types of foods you eat. Once foods are broken down into their component sugar parts, they can provide food for bacteria that cause tooth decay.

At one time, only the sugar sucrose was thought to be the food source for these bacteria. All sugars are now implicated, whether they are processed or natural. Sucrose, commonly consumed as brown or white sugar, is made up of fructose and glucose. Fructose is found in many fruits and honey; many cereals and grains as well as fruits and vegetables contain glucose. Lactose, another common sugar, is found in dairy products.

Your children should avoid frequent snacks that have a high content of simple sugars. This is also true of foods that adhere to the teeth for a prolonged time, like syrups and honey. Generally, complex carbohydrates, as contained in starchy foods, are less likely to cause tooth decay. Still, foods like pasta and starches such as potato can be the cause of cavities.

Good habits include limiting the frequency of carbohydrate or sugar intakes. Consuming a soft drink in a few minutes is less damaging to the teeth than continuously sipping it over an hour. Another practice is to limit the time that sticky foods are exposed to the teeth. Coconut syrup or dried candied mangos attach to the teeth more than coconut milk or fresh mangos. Have your children clean their teeth more often if they snack frequently or cannot follow these guidelines.

Disabled child needs preventive dentistry

We have a four-year-old child with a physical disability and
have difficulty cleaning her teeth. She can open her mouth but has
poor muscle coordination. How can we make brushing easier for her?

Have her visit your family dentist more frequently. A hygiene program could be set up specifically for your child, possibly involving prescription fluoride toothpaste or treatments with fluoride gels and rinses. These treatments can help control your daughter's increased risk for tooth decay.

Encourage your daughter, as much as possible, to clean her teeth to the best of her ability. She may have problems brushing and flossing, but understanding the need for cleaning is important. Children with disabilities often require dentists with special training to handle their unique physical and emotional needs and should start seeing a dentist within six months after their teeth begin to appear. Early visits are important to plan a preventive program to ensure good dental health.

Kids' untreated cavities become adult problems

Our six-year-old son has cavities in some of his back teeth. Since the teeth will be lost soon when his adult teeth come in, is it necessary to have them filled?

Baby Teeth Problems

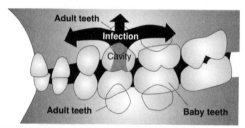

If baby tooth infections are not attended to, they could affect the development of adult teeth.

The health of baby teeth can directly affect your child's health and his developing adult teeth. Cavities are a form of infection. If the source of that infection is not removed, it may spread. The condition "rampant caries" refers to widespread decay in several teeth.

Infection in the teeth causes a structural breakdown which can make eating difficult and painful. In addition, weakened teeth are prone to fracture, which in turn make them more likely to cause traumatic injury to the surrounding gums and lips. Bacteria from infected teeth also may enter the bloodstream, causing potential problems to infants and children affected by other medical illnesses, particularly certain conditions of the heart. It also may increase the risk of mouth sores and throat infections.

Decayed teeth begin to break down and, in severe cases, are lost prematurely. With this loss, neighboring teeth begin to move out of position. There is thus a disruption in the pattern of normal growth. When infection spreads within a tooth, it often goes deep beneath the visible structure. Roots held by the jawbone become infected. If the infection spreads to these underlying areas, your child's adult teeth may become infected before they become visible.

These are good reasons for immediately attending to decay in a child's tooth.

There's no need to pull a decayed baby tooth

If a baby tooth is decayed, can it affect the adult tooth underneath? Should it be taken out?

The term decay refers to different degrees of infection. It can range from a small hole to complete destruction of the tooth above the gum. Only in severe cases is it necessary to extract the tooth. If the infection cannot be controlled by fillings or a root canal, removing the tooth will limit the risk of damage to the underlying adult tooth.

The baby teeth serve as spacers for adult teeth. If decay sets in to the baby tooth, it serves the adult tooth well to try to save the baby tooth with fillings or a root canal.

A deep infection penetrating the center of a baby tooth requires a pulpectomy, the equivalent of a root canal. Since decay in baby teeth responds better to treatment, a pulpotomy or partial root canal may be performed when the central portion of the nerve and blood supply is removed, leaving the roots untreated. In most cases, such procedures resolve severe infection in baby teeth.

It's not advisable to extract a baby tooth unless it can't be treated. Mobility of the tooth, with pain and pus draining from the gum around the tooth may also create a need for extraction. But saving baby teeth is important. They help maintain the space for adult teeth to come in properly. They also keep neighboring teeth from drifting inward toward the open space. Such movement may prevent normal eruption of underlying adult teeth. In such cases, tooth-spacers may be needed to keep teeth in their proper position.

Tooth removal is a last resort. Your dentist will do all that is necessary to keep teeth healthy. By doing so, it will insure your child's normal development of both teeth and jaws.

Baby Tooth Repair

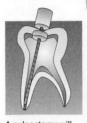 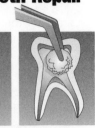

A pulpectomy will be done by using a file to remove the diseased pulp tissue.

The canals are dried with cotton pellets.

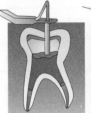 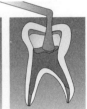

The canals are filled with a mixture.

Pressure is applied to the mixture.

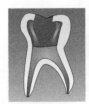 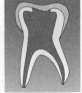

A pulpotomy only fills the top half of the tooth cavity.

A pulpectomy fills the tooth to the bottom of the roots. Then a stainless steel crown is added.

Sealants give teeth a shield from bacteria

My eight-year-old has no cavities.
Do you think she should have sealants to protect her teeth?

Yes and no. First, we will look at the disadvantages of using sealants in this situation. Your child has no cavities now, and unless her oral hygiene patterns, diet, or future permanent teeth change, and she becomes susceptible to tooth decay, she probably will continue to be cavity-free. Prevention can be maintained with regular checkups, good dental hygiene and a balanced diet.

Now let's look at some reasons why sealants might be preferred for your daughter. The procedure is simple and safe. It causes no harm to the teeth and prevents decay by inhibiting the collection of bacteria in areas where it may be difficult to clean.

Tooth Sealant

Tooth sealants are safe and provide 95% to 100% protection against decay. Here is how sealants are applied:

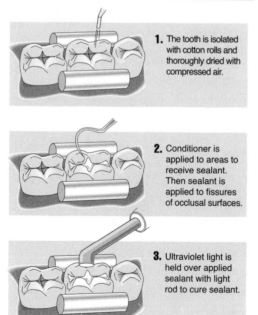

1. The tooth is isolated with cotton rolls and thoroughly dried with compressed air.

2. Conditioner is applied to areas to receive sealant. Then sealant is applied to fissures of occlusal surfaces.

3. Ultraviolet light is held over applied sealant with light rod to cure sealant.

The procedure is inexpensive. If a sealant saves a tooth from having a permanent filling, it may result in quite a savings. If the situation was changed and your daughter had several cavities, there would be little need for discussion; sealants would be strongly recommended. Sealants are described as the biggest advance in preventive dentistry since fluoride.

Sealants are plastic-like materials that are applied to the chewing surfaces of teeth. The material fills in the tiny pits and crevices where bacteria hide. Since the germs have fewer places to collect, decay in this area is prevented.

It's estimated that 80 percent of decay occurs on these biting surfaces. Studies show that with sealants, 95 to 100 percent of this decay can be eliminated.

Broken baby teeth may be fixed, but beware

Our two-year-old broke one of his front teeth after falling on the sidewalk. Our dentist recommended it be extracted, which we didn't want to do. Can fractured teeth be saved in these situations?

Many fractures of baby teeth can be saved. Restorative procedures using tooth-colored composite bonding materials can repair small defects. Larger fractures involving the nerve of the tooth may require treatment such as a root canal or crown. There are situations where extraction of the tooth is advisable. Your dentist has likely identified an existing or future problem that may cause complications later.

Most fractures to baby teeth can be repaired. But some of the types of fractures can cause problems to future permanent teeth. Here is how one repair is made:

Some injured teeth can later develop abscesses or cysts. If such a situation exists, your dentist is correct in advising removal of the tooth. Cysts and abscesses in baby teeth can affect and even prevent development of the underlying permanent teeth. In minor cases, alterations to the developing permanent tooth include discoloration and altered or incomplete crown formation. In severe cases, complete development of the adult tooth cannot continue and, eventually, the permanent tooth may require extraction.

Cracked Baby Teeth

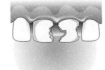
Damaged teeth

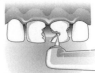
Decay is removed with a drill.

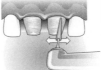
Approximately 1 to 1.5 mm of tooth structure is removed in a slightly tapered manner.

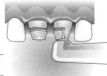
A V-shaped groove is formed to give attachment a solid anchor.

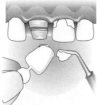
A composite material is placed into crown and is pushed into place with finger pressure.

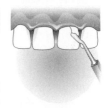
An excavator is used to remove excess material.

Extra teeth usually do not cause problems

My five-year-old has a tooth coming through his palate behind his two upper front teeth. It looks quite strange and now I'm concerned about his adult teeth coming in normally. What causes this? Will this cause a problem to his permanent teeth?

Removing Extra Teeth

Extra teeth growing in behind baby teeth can be unsightly, but don't usually threaten other teeth. This is how they can be removed surgically:

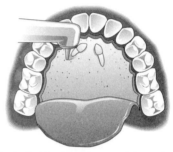

1. An incision is made around the teeth to expose the bone and protruding new teeth. A drill is used to uncover the teeth.

Extra teeth, referred to as supernumery, can appear at any age and almost any location in the mouth. Your son likely has a form referred to as a mesiodens. These are cone-shaped teeth with short roots that often appear between the upper front teeth. They usually cause no problems and developing permanent teeth can still come out normally. The cause is unknown.

Should a mesiodens not come out as part of normal tooth development, they may need to be extracted. Due to their unusual appearance and odd location, a mesiodens can be unsightly and concerning for parents.

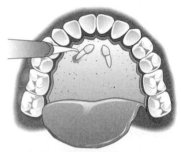

2. The teeth are then removed.

They can also be confused for premature erupting adult teeth. Such teeth can be extracted if parents are concerned with the appearance or if a mesiodens hinders any future tooth development.

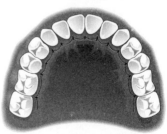

3. Sutures are then used to reattach the flap.

Swollen gums are common in kids with sickle cell anemia

Our one-year-old son has been diagnosed with sickle cell anemia by his pediatrician. He hasn't begun to teethe yet, but his gums are red and tender. Is the sickle cell anemia affecting his teeth?

Sickle cell anemia is a disease caused by deformed, oxygen-deficient, red blood cells that block small blood vessels in the body. In addition to many other problems, sickle cells are more fragile and may thus break more easily, causing internal bleeding problems.

It is a disease most common to peoples of African, Indian or Middle Eastern descent. Unfortunately, there remains no cure.

In children with sickle cell anemia, delayed tooth eruption and swelling of the gums are common. The red swelling in your son's mouth may indicate a sign of infection. You should have your dentist or pediatrician examine this area promptly. Parents must be warned that if an infection is present, especially in the mouth, the disease can escalate and develop into a severe viral infection involving fever, abdominal pain, lung complications, and if left untreated, death.

Sickle Cell Anemia

Sickle Cell Anemia usually occurs in people of African, Indian or Middle Eastern descent. It is the lack of oxygen in red blood cells causing them to deform into sickle shape. This in turn blocks smaller arteries.

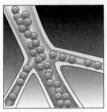

Regular red blood cells travel effortlessly through blood vessels.

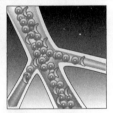

Oxygen starved sickle cells turn to sickle shapes and get caught on blood vessel walls.

Adults and children with sickle cell anemia must take special care in their oral hygiene habits to prevent any infections. Frequent teeth cleanings and fluoride treatments are of extreme importance. Antibiotics taken before certain dental procedures are advisable in some cases where possible infection may spread. Your dentist and physician will work together to establish a complete, thorough treatment regimen.

Space maintainers fill the void for adult teeth

Our seven-year-old son recently had a tooth extracted. Because it came out prematurely, the dentist said he would need a space maintainer. What is it?

Spacers for Teeth

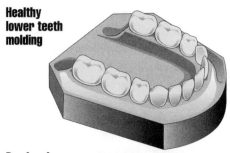

Healthy lower teeth molding

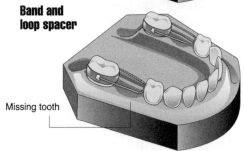

Band and loop spacer

Missing tooth

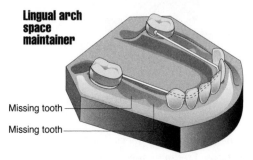

Lingual arch space maintainer

Missing tooth
Missing tooth

Space maintainers hold the space once occupied by a tooth. They consist of a metal band or cap that fits around the tooth on one side and a metal loop that extends over the gap and fits snugly against the tooth on the other side.

When a tooth is missing, a spacer can be used to replace it until an underlying permanent tooth erupts. Otherwise, the surrounding teeth can move out of position to fill the empty space.

Without a space maintainer, teeth near the space will shift and rotate out of position. Adult teeth may have insufficient room to erupt or may come in at awkward angles and positions. Space maintainers should be placed as soon as possible after the loss of a tooth and should be left in until the adult tooth begins to erupt.

Adults, too, can benefit from space maintainers if a fixed bridge cannot be placed in right away. If a permanent tooth is missing, space maintainers can keep surrounding teeth from moving. Failing to promptly restore a missing tooth or maintaining the space will result in the adjacent teeth angling inward toward the space.

Your dentist or orthodontist may then need to straighten and push the teeth back into position. Wearing a space maintainer may prevent more involved and costly orthodontic procedures.

Thumb sucking puts strain on teeth, palate

Our four-year-old has a habit of thumb sucking. We haven't been able to break him of the habit and are concerned about his teeth. What should we do?

Many psychologists believe that thumb sucking is normal. Unfortunately, it may lead to dental problems if continued for many years, especially after the age of seven when adult teeth begin to appear. The most common problem is protrusion of the upper front teeth. With constant pressure from the thumb, they may angle outward instead of growing straight down and may cause a change in appearance. Braces or orthodontic works are often needed to correct this.

A deeper or higher palate may be created by continual pressure from the thumb since bone is soft during the formative years. Breathing patterns may also be altered because of changes in the palate. Many mouth-breathing adults were thumb sucking children.

Thumb Sucking Damage

Although thumb sucking is normal, it may lead to dental problems in the later years. The most common problem can be the protrusion of the front teeth. Another can be the deepening of the upper palate.

Constant pressure from the thumb can cause the upper palate to deepen.

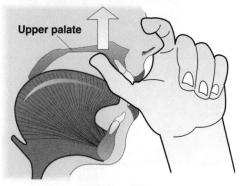

Upper palate

Thumb sucking

Thumb sucking may be a difficult habit to break. Parents should first try talking with the child. Help from a psychologist or dentist may also be needed. If these attempts fail, you may consider trying a mouth appliance specially designed to prevent thumb sucking. Any loss in the child's gratification from thumb sucking will be outweighed by the benefits of a healthier, more functional mouth.

Expanding child's jaw can give teeth room

Our daughter, who's now five, has teeth that are crowded and out of their normal position. The dentist said that her jaw is too small and that it needs an appliance to make it bigger. Is this type of treatment common and are there any problems that can develop from it?

It sounds more difficult than it is. But devices that expand a growing child's jaw can often give adult teeth the needed room to come in properly. Often, moving teeth can solve a crowded tooth problem.

Braces are the conventional method of moving teeth and are usually placed by an orthodontist. But if additional space is needed, something called an "expansion appliance" is used. It can either be attached to the teeth or be removable. Such appliances can be used on the upper or lower jaw.

The principle of these devices is the same. A spring or screw is attached to a plastic plate which acts on an area of the jaw, putting pressure on the underlying bone. The bone, in turn, molds to that pressure.

Removing Extra Teeth

Crowded teeth can be a problem for children with adult teeth coming in. Jaw expansion is one solution.

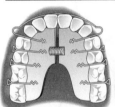 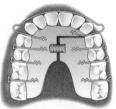

Screw in center is used to put lateral force to widen arch.

Screw is used to apply force to widen one side.

Through careful studies, specialists working with your family dentist can determine the proper amount of bone adjustments to enable normal alignment and function of the teeth and jawbone. Because the bone is easily moldable during childhood, these appliances only help to guide the bone in the desired way. By working with both variables of jaw size and tooth position, your dentist can often achieve a better final result.

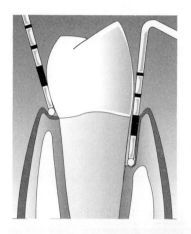

Chapter 4

Gum and Bone Health

Periodontics
- Perio (around) dontics (teeth)

Gum examination is vital for good oral health

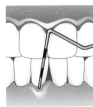

*Our family dentist recently poked and prodded
our gums to see how healthy they were.
He also did some tests that tells what bacteria are present.
Can you explain what these are for?
Also, why can't the dentist use x-rays to tell
how healthy the bone is around the teeth?*

Probing tips

As part of a dental examination, your dentist evaluates the health of your gums. Using a thin metal probe, he can measure certain areas around your teeth to see how healthy the bone support is around them.

Although x-rays show the amount of bone around the teeth, they limit the viewer to a general understanding. Probe measurements allow the dentist to identify problem areas around teeth that may seem normal visually and on the x-ray.

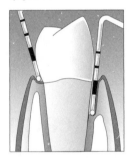

*The probe on the left side of the tooth shows
healthy bones and gums. The probe on the
right shows gums that need treatment.*

Because gum disease is so prevalent, especially in adults more than 30 years of age, routine checks of your gum health are important. Bacterial detection tests can identify gum problems. Treated paper strips are placed in areas around the gums to help identify the bacteria present. Certain bacteria and enzymes are known to be associated with gum disease. These can be identified and used as a diagnostic tool in identifying potential disease areas.

Surgery is unnecessary with good hygiene

*After I finished my dental cleaning, the hygienist and dentist
recommended that I have a procedure called "root planing"
and "curettage." Can you explain what these are?*

Healthy gums and teeth require only routine cleanings. When infection of the gums and bone, termed periodontitis, creates a pocket of gum tissue around the teeth, trapping bacterial deposits, special attention is required. Root planing and curettage are advanced forms of the tooth-cleaning process and often require the use of local anesthetic.

Specialized hand instruments are used to smooth root surfaces, ridding them of deposits. The instrument tips are shaped to allow cleaning beneath the gumline.

Root planing is the removal of bacterial collections of plaque and calculus (calcified deposits) from the roots of the teeth. In gingival curettage, the inner surface of the gum cuff that surrounds the tooth is removed.

Root Planing

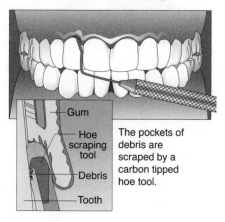

Root planing is a cleaning of tooth pocket-debris from between gum and tooth.

Gum

Hoe scraping tool

Debris

Tooth

The pockets of debris are scraped by a carbon tipped hoe tool.

Acute conditions such as gum abscesses can be treated by combining these procedures and use of antibiotics. Root planing and curettage may also be effective in treating advanced gum diseases where other surgical procedures are not advisable. For example, patients with severe medical illnesses may not be able to tolerate more serious gum surgery.

Because root planing and curettage have been recommended, you should be more conscious of good oral hygiene. Proper care and regular checkups can help you avoid more complicated gum surgery.

Exposing the causes of sensitive teeth

My upper back teeth are sensitive by the gumline when I brush my teeth or have a cold drink. After using a special toothpaste for sensitive teeth, the sensitivity still remains. What causes this and how can it be relieved?

Sensitivity of teeth at the gumline often results from an exposed root surface. Gums normally cover the roots, but many people have receding gums, exposing this otherwise protected area.

Vigorous brushing and bite problems also can cause tooth sensitivity, even in people who do not suffer from receding gums. Other sources of root sensitivity include prolonged exposure to sweet and sour foods and drinks, and various dental procedures, such as extensive tooth cleanings, extractions, fillings and gum surgeries.

There are many degrees of sensitivity and various treatment options to relieve the discomfort. Special toothpastes are commonly used for slight cases of discomfort. Both products are available without a prescription. A variety of solutions can also be applied by your dentist to relieve persistent sensitivity; concentrated fluorides are widely used. Your dentist may apply agents that block tiny tubules in the exposed tooth areas that are related to the sensitivity. In severe cases, a filling may be needed to guard the nerve at the core of the tooth and its roots.

Any prolonged and unusual sensitivity should be reported to your dentist. Prompt attention will usually provide a safe and effective solution.

Bone loss can leave root gaps prone to infection

A gum specialist has told me that some of my back teeth will be hard to clean because of furcations. Can you tell me exactly what these are and why it is harder to clean teeth with them?

Furcation refers to the space between the roots of teeth that have lost bone support. A furcation involves teeth with more than one root. Normally, the roots of teeth are firmly anchored in bone so that only the crown or portion normally above the gumline is exposed. However, when gum disease spreads, the level of bone and/or gums may leave areas between roots infected and cause bone loss.

If furcations are found in some of your back teeth, efforts are made to clean these areas. Often, gum surgery is needed to lower the height of your gums that

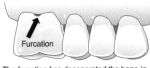

Furcation

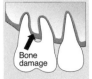

Bone damage

The furcation has degenerated the bone in this cutaway.

may cover up these hidden spaces. By exposing the spaces, you may be better able to clean them with special brushes and flosses.

If left untreated, an infection in a furcation area will result in the continued loss of bone between the roots. Regular brushing and flossing will not help clean these areas.

There is usually little or no pain from infected furcations. However, once one is discovered by your dentist, you should carefully follow instructions and procedures needed to control ongoing infection. Gum surgery and special cleanings can help resolve a furcation problem that, without treatment, can eventually cause tooth loss.

Loose teeth are a warning of gum, bone trouble

Several of my husband's teeth recently became
loose for no apparent reason. Can something
be done to strengthen them?

Dental procedures can strengthen loose teeth
in some cases, depending on the cause. Reversible
problems include premature contact between
one or more teeth when you bite. Normally, teeth
fit together in a way that evenly distributes pressure.
When biting places undue stress on a tooth or small group of teeth,
they can loosen. Correcting the bite with crowns or bridges or by adjusting the
height of the premature contact area often strengthens loose teeth.

Habits such as lip and cheek biting or chewing on a pencil can force
teeth out of position. Likewise, pipe smoking and even playing certain wind
instruments can put stress on incisors or front teeth. If these actions are
stopped or controlled, teeth can be strengthened.

Gum and bone disease, or periodontitis, is the single most common cause
of loose teeth. Infection around the teeth causes the supporting structures to
break down. As bone and gum support diminish, so does the tooth's ability to
withstand the stress of normal eating. Continued infection may result in loss of
teeth. Splinting or joining of the teeth with a wire brace along with bonding
material can help increase their strength, but continual home care and
professional cleanings are needed. Loose teeth are a warning sign. Prompt
attention may help prevent tooth loss.

Gum recession isn't uncommon in youth

I'm only 16 and already my dentist tells me that my gums are receding.
Doesn't this usually happen to older people?
What can I do to prevent further recession?

Gum recession is common among younger people
in the United States and in northern European countries
where good oral hygiene is practiced. Excessive
and rigorous brushing especially along the gumline
is a common cause of gum recession.

Gingival recession occurs when the attachment
of gum tissue to the teeth breaks down. After this

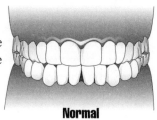

Normal

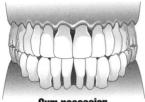

Gum recession

Receding gums usually can be attributed to neglect in oral hygiene and sometimes to vigorous brushing. It can also be caused by muscle tension on the gums or crowns that extend into the gumline irritating the gums.

happens, the root surfaces of the teeth normally covered by the gums become exposed. Aside from being aesthetically displeasing, these exposed root surfaces are now prone to decay.

There may be other associated causes of receding gums. For example, muscle attachments called frenum may pull excessively on an area of gum tissue. Crowns that extend around the tooth deep into the gums may irritate the surrounding tissue. Even the way that the teeth emerge into the mouth may place an increased risk for future recession.

Once the tissue has receded, medications can be applied to rid the sensitivity. To prevent further recession caused by incorrect brushing, proper oral hygiene instructions should be given. Your dentist will evaluate specific treatments for other problems causing the recession.

Poor oral care adds to midterm blues

Last week, after studying for a midterm exam, I noticed my gums were puffy and painful. My roommate commented that I had bad breath. Could this be caused by stress?

Your symptoms describe a condition known as ANUG, or acute necrotizing ulcerative gingivitis. It is also called Vincent's infection or more commonly "trench mouth."

Although the causes are not completely understood, poor oral hygiene and fatigue or stress is commonly associated with this disorder. The chances are increased if you are a smoker because tar tends to irritate the gums. Stress alone is unlikely to be the cause, but neglect of oral hygiene is likely during the stressful period before exams. Poor diet and health also increase the risk of gum infection.

Visit your dentist promptly, even if your immediate symptoms pass. Without professional care, the condition could recur or develop into a more serious condition, "periodontitis ulcerosa." A thorough cleaning of gums and teeth is the first step in treatment. Antibiotic rinses or ointments, as well as hydrogen-peroxide rinses, are commonly prescribed to help fight infection. In more serious cases, antibiotic pills may be recommended.

A dark blue spot on gums just an amalgam tattoo

I've noticed a small, dark blue spot on my gums.
It doesn't hurt, but it won't go away. What is it?

In most cases, small, dark blue spots on gums are a result of silver amalgam deposits. If the gum is scraped during the placement of a silver filling, the silver or mercury in the filling stains the protein portion of the gums. The spot is called an amalgam tattoo. It is a permanent stain and poses no complications. These tattoos do not require treatment and should be excised only if you are over-concerned with its appearance.

There are certain colored spots that can lead to more serious outcomes. Although these are rare, they should not be overlooked. Should a spot ever change in size or color, you should promptly have it checked. Such changes warrant concern.

Part of your regular dental checkup includes detection of such spots and growths. Although most are normal and pose no risks, some can be serious and involve surgery. Regular checkups avoid such ongoing and developing problems.

Electrosurgery offers an alternative to the knife

My dentist wants to remove a piece of excess gum tissue with
a procedure he calls "electrosurgery." The name makes me nervous.
Can you explain what this is?

Electrosurgery, or radiosurgery, uses radio waves to separate cell or soft-tissue layers in the mouth. No electric current is involved, despite the name. The procedure is commonly used to remove or modify parts of the gum, cheek or other soft tissues in the mouth. It is used in combination with or as a substitute for cutting with a scalpel or other sharp instrument. Radio waves are generated through a control box and sent to a hand piece which the dentist applies to the affected area. The intensity of the

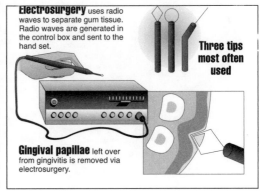

Electrosurgery uses radio waves to separate gum tissue. Radio waves are generated in the control box and sent to the hand set.

Three tips most often used

Gingival papillae left over from gingivitis is removed via electrosurgery.

waves is carefully controlled so that only certain areas of tissue are affected.

Radiosurgery has some advantages: bleeding is more easily controlled and less scar tissue may be formed during the healing. It is also easier to work in hard-to-reach places with this device. If you choose electrosurgery, be aware that the reaction of the instrument to tissue may create a strong burning odor.

Grafting of gum tissue can end a recession

Our daughter has a lower tooth with gum recession. It doesn't hurt, but quite a bit of the root of the tooth shows, and she's self conscious about smiling. Is there anything that can be done?

There are several causes for gum recession on isolated teeth. Muscle attachments from the lips can create a tension on an area of the gums, pulling them away. Tartar and plaque accumulation as a constant irritant is associated with recession. Abrasion from over vigorous tooth brushing also leads to gum recession.

Grafting Gums

Sometimes receding gums can be attributed to tension along the gumline. This blanching of the gums can be corrected with grafting.

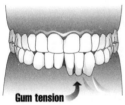

Gum tension

Tension along the gumline pulls at the gums and causes a recession. An incision will be made (arrow) to loosen the tension.

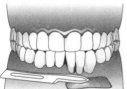

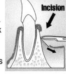

The incision is made just below the problem area. The lip and cheek naturally pull the wound open and the gum tension is released.

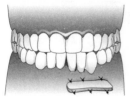

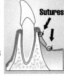

A gum graft is retrieved from the roof of the mouth and sutured into the wound. It should take 7 or 8 days for the graft to heal.

Grafting healthy gum tissue from one area of the mouth to another area affected by recession can help to maintain normal gum appearance and restore tissue health. There are many techniques for grafting tissue, depending on the types of defects. The procedure is often safe, simple and effective in repairing a diseased or traumatized gum area.

Your daughter may require two types of grafting procedures depending on how much recession she has. The first graft helps prevent further recession by placing new tissue which can attach to the underlying bone around the tooth. The recession is still noticeable after this treatment, but further recession is halted. After one to two years, a second grafting procedure repositions the gum tissue at a normal height to match surrounding teeth and gums.

A general dentist or periodontist, a gum specialist, can perform grafting procedures. Success of the treatment depends on the degree and location of the recession and on the health of your gums and the bone surrounding the tooth. Often, preliminary procedures like tooth cleaning and minor gum surgery are needed to ensure a successful graft.

Special "shield" helps heal diseased gums

My husband's gum specialist recommended using Gore-Tex material to treat his gum disease. What is this and how does it work?

Gore-Tex, derived from Teflon, has proven invaluable as a mending material for blood vessels. Dentists have begun using the material to help diseased gum and bone tissue regenerate.

As infection around a tooth progresses, the gum tissue that normally helps support the tooth starts to pull away. Infected bone around the tooth also deteriorates, often causing the tooth to become loose. In advanced cases, the loss is often irreversible.

Membranes made from Gore-Tex protect uninfected gum tissue from infected tissue while antibiotics heal the areas

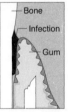

Infected area is surgically removed.

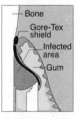

The Gore-Tex shield is added between infected area and uninfected tissue.

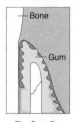

The Gore-Tex shield is removed after bone and gum tissue has regenerated.

But infection can be eliminated and controlled. A dentist may attempt to clean out the bacteria through surgery to allow healthy tissue to reform. Membranes such as Gore-Tex acts as a shield, keeping infected tissue away during the healing process and allowing the formation of tiny fibers in the gums that hold the tooth in place. Artificial bone may be used in conjunction with gum surgery to restore the original bone support around the tooth.

Healing takes four to six weeks, and during this time, the membrane will be removed. As long as you can be careful to clean the area after treatment, your tooth will likely have a second chance.

Women's hormones are linked to gum disease

*I take care of my teeth and gums more than my husband,
and still the dentist tells me that my gums are not as healthy as his.
Are there any differences between men and women that
make it more difficult for women to control gum problems?*

Pregnancy Gingivitis

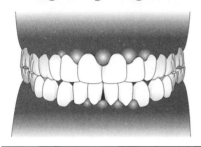

*Pregnancy, and the hormone
activity that goes with it, can
cause a high level of the hormone
progesterone that has been
associated with gum inflammation*

Changes in hormonal levels during puberty, menstruation, pregnancy and menopause are linked to gum problems. Although good oral hygiene is a primary factor in maintaining healthy gums, hormonal changes for women can confuse and frustrate even diligent dental care efforts. However, being aware of the association can help women predict and control such influences.

During puberty, high levels of the hormone progesterone are associated with gum inflammation. Likewise, menstruation may be linked to gingivitis and even cold sores in some women. Oral contraceptives are another important influencing dental factor for women. They can be linked to dry mouths, pigmentation on the gums and gingivitis.

The estrogen component or oral contraceptives can affect blood clotting in some women. Thus, certain oral surgeries may have an additional complication of prolonged bleeding. In addition, oral contraceptives will often not work if antibiotics used in dental treatment are prescribed.

Hormone changes in pregnancy are associated with gum inflammation that has been appropriately named "pregnancy gingivitis." And the final hormone changes of menopause have been linked to everything from dry mouth and a burning sensation of the tongue to receding gums.

The association of hormone changes and dental disease is important to understand. Proper treatment can be reinforced better if such effects are known. For example, a pregnant woman may think swollen gums are a temporary condition. However, if neglected, this alteration may result in an ongoing gum problem.

As a general rule, be persistent in your oral hygiene efforts. Don't let hormonal changes frustrate your ongoing care. In addition, let your dentist know about such changes since they may be linked to some of your dental problems.

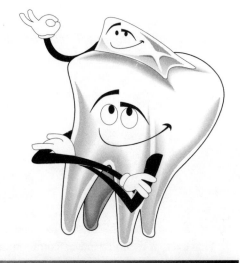

Chapter 5

Cavities and Fillings
Restorative Dentistry

Weight of new filling is worth a pound of cure

My dentist wants to replace several of my old fillings.
They aren't decayed and don't feel sensitive. Can I wait another year
since my dental insurance will cover a higher percentage of the fees?

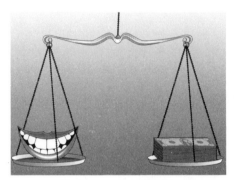

The type of dental restoration and when it is performed is often limited by insurance guidelines and benefits. Some dental plans will not pay your dentist to perform certain procedures. Other plans will pay an increasing percentage of the service the longer you are a member. Economically, a match between payment of benefits and timing of treatment would be ideal.

However, you should never compromise the benefits of needed dental treatment or even the risk of not completing a preventive service in order to minimize your cost. Although silver amalgam is a good filling material, old fillings may need to be replaced after many years.

During your regular checkups, your dentist and hygienist will point out old fillings that may have evidence of decay around them. Your dentist also may suggest that other fillings which are worn, cracked or at risk of being decayed, be replaced. Because an area of decay is so small, it often can go undetected in an x-ray. Usually, by the time you feel any discomfort in a tooth with an existing filling, it may indicate a more complicated and costly procedure.

Sensitivity to cold is a phase of recovery

My dentist recently put a gold filling in one of my teeth and

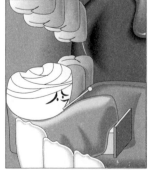

it's sensitive when I drink cold water.
Will this ever go away?

Most likely yes. Placement of large metal fillings may bring about temporary tooth sensitivity. The most common cause is the trauma of drilling and cleaning out deep decay. After the work is done, the tooth goes through a healing state referred to as "hyperemia," the increased blood flow that occurs in a site that has been traumatized. Cold sensitivity is a sign of this recovery phase.

Usually, over a period of weeks, cold sensitivity will lessen. An increase in pain or a sensitivity to both hot and cold indicates trouble healing. The trauma of removing deep decay can disrupt a tooth's healing mechanism, making a root canal necessary.

Device caps the risk of infection to nerves

Because my cavity was deep, my dentist said he
needed to put a pulp cap underneath it. What does this do?
What would happen if just the filling was put in without the pulp cap?

A pulp cap is placed in a cavity which has extensive decay. The area of infection in such cases is close to the nerve and blood supply, or pulp, of the tooth. A protective pulp cap layer is placed over the area of the underlying nerve before the final filling is completed. Pulp cap material is made up of calcium hydroxide, the same components as your natural teeth.

Pulp Cap

A pulp cap is placed in a cavity which has
extensive decay. It protects the blood supply
and nerve or pulp from infection.

Filling

Calcium hydroxide pulp cap

Tooth

Root

Pulp

There are two reasons for placing a pulp cap in a deep cavity. The first is to help the area around the nerve to heal. The second is to insulate the nerve and blood supply from temperature changes. Metal fillings placed over the pulp cap layer can conduct significant temperature changes. Without a pulp cap, a tooth may be sensitive to hot and particularly cold liquids. In more extreme cases, nerve damage may result.

When a pulp cap is needed, the dentist will inform you of a risk to a potentially damaged or infected pulp. In some cases, additional treatment is needed if a tooth cannot recover with a pulp cap and filling. Persistent sensitivity to temperature changes and/or a spontaneous dull ache after a deep filling has been placed may indicate permanent nerve damage.

Silver amalgam fillings pose no health threat

I've read that silver amalgam fillings are related to certain health problems including multiple sclerosis and liver disease. Should I consider having my fillings replaced with something better to avoid the risks of these health problems?

Silver amalgam fillings are safe, effective and supported strongly by the American Dental Association. Dentists place 100 million amalgam fillings in teeth each year in the United States. With the exception of a few allergies and unproven medical risks, silver amalgams have an excellent safety record. As for the association to multiple sclerosis, experts from the National Multiple Sclerosis Society refute any link.

The controversy focuses on the mercury content of silver amalgam, usually about 50 percent. Although mercury is toxic at high levels, the metal in dental amalgam is inactive. In combination with components such as copper, tin, and silver, the mercury becomes biologically safe. Mercury vapor can escape in tiny amounts during vigorous chewing but there is no evidence to associate this with toxic effects. The American Dental Association strictly advises against the removal of dental amalgams for health reasons not related to an allergy.

How common are allergies to mercury? Approximately 50 cases of allergic reactions have been reported since 1905. Silver amalgams have worked well during the 150 years they've been used in America.

Dentists go for gold when tooth gets old

Inlay   Onlay   Crown

My lower back tooth will have a gold onlay filling. Is there also a filling called an inlay? Which is better and why is one recommended over another?

Gold restorations fall into several categories depending on the amount of coverage of the tooth by gold. The most common types include inlay, onlay and crown.

An inlay usually has its borders within the confines of the biting surface of a tooth. An onlay usually extends beyond the biting surfaces. When the extent of coverage goes to the gumline on the front or back of the tooth, the restoration is often classified as a type of crown.

A dentist recommends gold restorations based on the amount of tooth surfaces that need to be protected and repaired. The choice is balanced on one side by conserving healthy tooth structure and on the other side by limiting any future tooth fracture that might occur because of insufficient coverage.

Your dentist considers factors such as biting force, unusual or unnatural contact with the teeth when closing and ongoing tooth decay in selecting the restoration that best fits your needs.

Temporary fillings may halt infection's spread

My dentist wants to place temporaries in several of my teeth, then begin working on permanent fillings. Why doesn't he just start doing permanent fillings one tooth at a time?

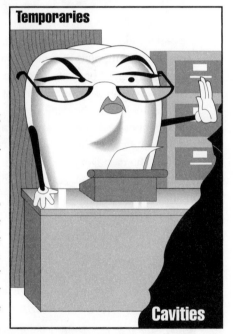

Your dentist is practicing something called caries control. When a dentist sees a person that has many cavities, his or her first priority is to control the disease. Cavities are the result of a bacterial infection that can spread not only to other parts of your mouth, but to the mouths of others. Several studies have described how mothers transmit bacteria from their teeth to their infants. By controlling the infection with temporary fillings, your dentist can remove the source of the ongoing infection.

Since permanent fillings may take months to complete, your dentist has elected to prevent further tooth decay. A small cavity at the onset could increase in size, and a larger cavity could result in an infection that requires root canal treatment.

Temporaries placed during caries control are usually made of mild healing ingredients that are strong enough to keep bacteria from entering the tooth. Teeth with temporaries can often be worked on months later, with no additional decay or damage suffered during the repair period.

Failed filling doesn't signal incompatibility

My temporary filling came out. This is the second time and now I'm nervous that the permanent one won't last. Why does the temporary keep coming out and does this indicate possible problems when the permanent one is completed?

Pliable Temporary

Permanent
Metallic Filling

Various techniques and materials are used in making temporary fillings. Techniques vary with cements that harden in the filling space and materials such as acrylic resins that are molded to fit an area, then cemented.

The choice of temporary material and the technique used depend on the size and location of the decayed or restored area. Smaller holes can usually be filled with a temporary cement, while larger areas need to be covered and protected by metal or plastic temporary crowns. Temporaries, as their name implies, are only meant to protect and last for a short time until more permanent work can be done.

A temporary can come out for a variety of reasons. Hard abrasive foods and moisture contamination are some factors which can cause a temporary to dislodge. The dislodging of a temporary crown will not predict the outcome of a permanent restoration. Permanent fillings are custom made to fit the teeth so any moisture problems are avoided.

Structurally, permanent restorations are made of stronger materials and held in place by cements which can withstand biting and chewing forces.

Starting at the back helps teeth in front

When I went to the dentist he wanted to start working on my back teeth first. Would you please explain why?

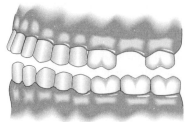

Your dentist is concerned with structure and function in choosing to start with your back teeth. He or she has set a well-founded priority for your care. Your back teeth are critical in maintaining the vertical dimension of your jaw and determining how your teeth meet when you bite. Without these structural pillars, your front teeth would undergo considerable stress.

Over time, a person who loses several back teeth without seeking dental care will experience teeth shifting. The front teeth will often flare out. Why? Since there are fewer teeth in the back of the mouth to help guide the bite, the front teeth assume this role. They are not intended to withstand this stress and respond by gradually flaring out.

If you are concerned with the appearance of some of your front teeth, let your dentist know. There may be an easy way to temporarily repair them. When faced with structural, functional and aesthetic considerations at the same time, your dentist is correct in placing priority on structure and function.

Glass ionomer fillings help the cavity prone

Our seven-year-old girl has had a lot of cavities. Recently, our family dentist has started putting something called "glass ionomer" in her fillings. Why does he use this instead of the silver that he uses for our older boy?

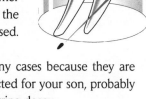

Glass ionomer is an old material that has recently regained popularity. It has some characteristics which, for your daughter, may make it the material of choice. Since she has several cavities, simply replacing decayed areas with silver or amalgam fillings may not keep bacteria from spreading around those same areas. Glass ionomer contains a glass-like powder that has fluoride. Once the material is in the mouth, the fluoride is slowly released. This fluoride helps prevent further decay.

Silver amalgam fillings are still preferred in many cases because they are stronger and often last longer. This material was selected for your son, probably because he doesn't suffer the same problem of recurring decay.

Glass ionomers have additional uses as well. They are often used as protective insulating layers for deep fillings. Used as sealants, these compounds prevent decay from getting into the cracks and fissures of newly erupted permanent teeth. Because glass ionomers stick to the teeth, no potentially harmful solutions, such as those used in bonding, need to be applied. However, they are not as tooth-like in appearance as the bonding materials, and are often not as strong.

Posts put the bite back in badly damaged teeth

My father recently had a metal post placed in one of his teeth. Why? Is it safe?

Metal posts are usually placed in teeth that have been badly broken down. They act as additional support in building back the area of a tooth decayed or missing. Posts are cemented in one or more roots of a tooth after a root canal procedure is completed. Because they are firmly anchored inside the roots of the teeth, posts act as a strong foundation to rebuild teeth.

For teeth broken off at the gumline, a post may be the only way to restore or save a tooth. Composite bonding materials or metals are attached to the post to build up the area; a crown may then be used to restore the tooth.

Posts can be either custom made or pre-made to fit various root lengths and diameters. Likewise, posts are made of many materials including gold, stainless steel and titanium. Some people have reported allergies to stainless steel, so titanium alloys and gold may be safer.

Tooth Posts

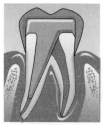

Post and core to add height to the crown preparation.

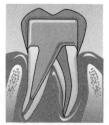

Post and core with a coping to replace coronal tooth structure.

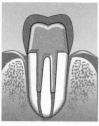

Two parallel posts and core.

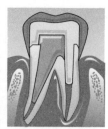

Two separate posts with interlocking cores.

The rebuilding of a tooth after loss near the gumline can be done with a post added to the base of the tooth. Here are a few different types of posts:

Posts do present slight risks. Drills used to prepare the hole into which a post will fit can perforate the root and open an area to possible infection. Chewing stress to the post also may cause root fracture and eventual tooth loss. However, the benefits of being able to save and restore a tooth outweigh the risks.

Cavities become more prevalent in the elderly

Why am I getting more cavities at the age of 67?
I thought after a certain age, cavities were not a problem.

That statement was true 20 years ago, but trends in tooth decay are changing. As a rule, tooth decay had been the most prevalent dental disease for those under the age of 30. For people older than 30, gum disease was the overriding concern. While that generality still holds for many, conditions like yours are more common.

Recent studies suggest that people in their 60s and 70s can have as many as 40 percent more cavities than those in their 20s and 30s. Many elderly people take medications that may interfere with or prevent saliva secretion. Without saliva, one of the body's defenses against tooth decay, teeth become more prone to cavities.

In addition, older people now retain more of their teeth than ever before. Dentures are becoming less common, and natural teeth are functioning longer. Although these retained teeth help considerably in daily life, they are still prone to decay from such factors as medications. Radiation therapy in cancer patients also leads to increased tooth decay because salivary glands are compromised during treatment.

To help prevent further decay, good oral hygiene, use of fluorides and regular visits to your dentist are advisable. Sometimes changing medications that hinder saliva secretion may be helpful.

Different drills are used for different tasks

The last time I had a filling done, my dentist used a drill that vibrated so much it hurt. Why didn't he just keep using the first high-pitched one that's normally used?

There are two broad categories of dental drills. In the first are high speed drills that rotate at several hundred thousand rpms. These are used for cutting through teeth and metal. They are water-cooled to prevent overheating of the teeth.

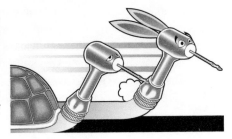

In the second category are low speed drills that rotate less than 100,000 rpms. Cleaning areas of tooth decay is an example of a chore for this slower handpiece. Low speed drills are also used for polishing teeth and fillings.

Because the two drills work at such different speeds, each has its own characteristics. The high speed drill often feels painless since it cuts so easily and rapidly. Low speed drills cause the teeth to vibrate more but are actually less traumatic. Low speed drills usually do not require water cooling since the heat created is moderate and easily controlled. Your dentist selects the type of drill used based on the difficulty of the cutting chore and by the goal of limiting the amount of heat trauma to the teeth involved.

"Splints" help keep loose teeth in place

My dentist joined my lower front teeth together with
bonding material. He said that would help them last longer.

How does this work?

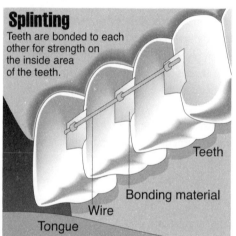

Splinting

Teeth are bonded to each other for strength on the inside area of the teeth.

Teeth

Bonding material

Wire

Tongue

Teeth compromised by gum and bone disease often become loose due to loss of supporting bone anchoring the teeth in your jaw. Chewing aggravates this condition and may cause teeth to be prematurely lost.

"Splinting" is the process of joining teeth together to reinforce and stabilize a loose tooth. Splinting is also used to stabilize teeth loosened in accidents. Bonding material or composite resins can be used to bind teeth, or a wire can be fitted across the inside surfaces of the teeth. Teeth that are capped or crowned also can be splinted. Often two or more teeth are joined with cast gold or porcelain bridgework.

Although splinting is an effective short-term solution, there are long-term disadvantages. Joining teeth with bonding, for example, creates areas that become more difficult to clean. Unless these areas are flossed daily, further infection may increase the chances of bone loss. This could also result in tooth loss. The procedure is effective only if proper hygiene is followed.

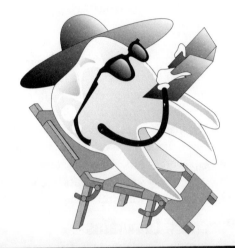

Chapter 6

Esthetics
Cosmetic Dentistry

Painless techniques result in whiter teeth

I've always wanted whiter teeth. Is there an easy way to lighten them without having to put crowns on my teeth? And, can strong sunlight affect the color?

Yes, you can have whiter teeth. Besides the more conventional bonding of teeth, where plastic materials are layered over problem areas, your dentist can place porcelain coverings on the teeth or bleach them. Both techniques are painless, usually done without local anesthetic, and are considerably less expensive than crowns. The porcelain coverings are custom designed shells that fit over the teeth. Tooth-bleaching is done with chemicals and light, and involves several visits. The porcelain shells and tooth-bleaching have five or more years of successful track records and can provide you some new options to explore with your dentist.

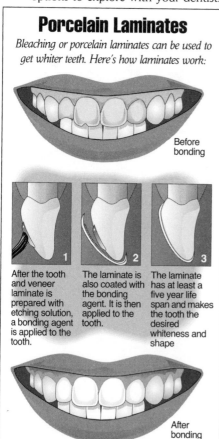

Porcelain Laminates

Bleaching or porcelain laminates can be used to get whiter teeth. Here's how laminates work:

Before bonding

1 After the tooth and veneer laminate is prepared with etching solution, a bonding agent is applied to the tooth.

2 The laminate is also coated with the bonding agent. It is then applied to the tooth.

3 The laminate has at least a five year life span and makes the tooth the desired whiteness and shape

After bonding

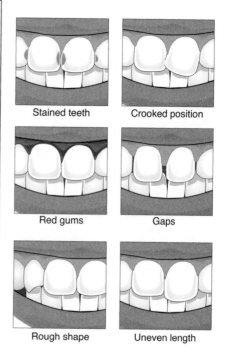

Stained teeth

Crooked position

Red gums

Gaps

Rough shape

Uneven length

In answer to your second question, sunlight can be useful in maintaining color after bleaching treatment. Smiling in the sunshine, however, probably won't change your tooth color.

Simple surgery can correct unsightly gaps

I have a space between my front two teeth that looks terrible.
What causes this and what can I do to fix it?

Spaces or diastemas can occur any-where in the mouth, although they appear more frequently in the upper front teeth. Habits like lip-biting, tongue-thrusting and finger or thumb pressure may play an early role in forcing teeth apart. Missing teeth or hereditary factors, like large jaws with comparatively small teeth, can also cause unnatural spacing. A muscle attachment called a frenum may also put undue stress on teeth, causing them to shift position.

Gaps in the teeth or "diastemas" usually occur in the upper front teeth. Often these gaps require orthodontics to correct. Some gaps are candidates for tooth bonding.

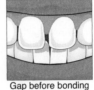 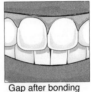

Gap before bonding procedure   Gap after bonding procedure

Besides the often displeasing appearance, spaces may affect speech patterns, with consonant sounds changing according to the degree of air flow between the teeth. Eating habits, particularly biting, are also affected.

Dentists treat diastemas according to the cause or causes which created the space. Habits like thumb-sucking often require orthodontics to correct the pressures that originally forced the teeth out of position. Hereditary factors are difficult to treat. In the case of missing teeth, prosthetic devices like bridges need to be made to restore spaces where teeth normally would appear.

If the space is between your two front teeth and is relatively small, a simple procedure like tooth bonding is often adequate. Tooth-colored materials are mechanically and chemically attached to a tooth surface changing its width, length or overall appearance.

Simple surgical procedures can correct spaces caused by a frenum, by relieving stress that forces teeth apart. However, certain cases require more costly and involved procedures that may provide you with a more natural and long-lasting result.

Crack lines in teeth are normally harmless

I have noticed vertical crack lines on the outer surface of my front tooth. My girlfriend doesn't have them.
How do these form and can they be removed?

Cracks, or "crazing," usually result from accidental blows to the front teeth. If you've always noticed the cracks and are experiencing no pain or sensitivity, don't worry. Craze lines can also form from biting pressure or a sudden temperature change.

Most of us have these cracks; the number varies depending on the strength and thickness of your tooth enamel and on your eating or biting habits. The cracks are easier to see in translucent or dark teeth.

Cracks sometimes are the first sign of a fracture. If a tooth is sensitive to pressure or cold food, visit your dentist promptly. These symptoms may indicate that a fracture line extends into the deeper layers of a tooth.

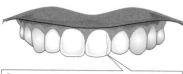

Craze cracks can occur on teeth that have experienced accidental blows or from biting pressure. The degree of the crack can be determined by a dentist.

Your dentist can perform tests to determine the extent of a crack. Among them is a "vitality test" in which a pencil-like probe is used to gauge the health of the pulp and nerve within the tooth.

Porcelain coverings called laminates, or bonding, can be used to mask these lines for cosmetic purposes.

Rough tooth surfaces are prone to stains

My 17-year-old daughter has teeth that are beginning to turn yellow. The color change began two years ago and is getting worse, especially around the edges of her teeth. She had braces five years ago and bonding eight to ten years ago. Can you tell us the cause?

If you have only recently noticed the stains, the most likely cause is the accumulation of stains on the bonded areas. Over time, bonded surfaces can

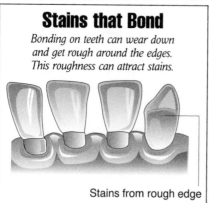

Stains that Bond

Bonding on teeth can wear down and get rough around the edges. This roughness can attract stains.

Stains from rough edge

become rough, making them more prone to staining by foods. The areas most vulnerable are the edges where the composite filling ends and the tooth begins. Frequently, the bond between tooth and filling will break, allowing stained material to be retained.

Staining can become worse with polishing by a hygienist or brushing with an abrasive toothpaste. Such action can further roughen the surface of the bonding material.

Another possibility is inadequate brushing or infrequent fluoride treatments during the time your daughter wore braces. Teeth require a thorough cleaning and a regular fluoride supplement program since braces make cleaning more difficult.

Chronic stains should be evaluated by a physician if dental causes have been checked and eliminated. Let both your general dentist and orthodontist know of your concern so that a more detailed evaluation can be made.

Many factors color the choice of a crown's hue

One of the crowns on my front teeth doesn't quite match the color of the others. I didn't notice it so much after my dentist put it in, but now it bothers me. What could cause this?

The color of teeth is both subtle and complex. Many factors determine the color of a tooth. Shades may range from a brownish orange to white with wide variations in between. In addition, some teeth are more opaque while others are more transparent. Even the relative brightness of a tooth is variable. To make matters more complex, these factors are variable depending on the area of a tooth by the gumline as compared to the biting edge.

Your dentist takes many of these factors into account when describing the color to the ceramicist who will make the crown. Porcelain shades usually are selected from samples that closely resemble your tooth. Any deviation from the sample then is described so that some of the subtlety that defines your tooth can be reproduced.

Teeth can change in color over time while porcelain color will remain relatively constant. The color change you now notice may be due to several factors. The brightness of the light, the type of light (e.g., natural versus fluorescent) and what colors were surrounding the immediate area of the new porcelain crown are all important in your perception of the color.

When your dentist describes a color, daylight or a color-correcting light are the most accurate and constant light sources and a "Grey Card," used by photographers, is the most neutral background on which to view the color. Otherwise, the color you view in one setting may not match when you see the crown in a different light or surrounding.

There can be factors beyond the control of your dentist since color is so complex. Because the perception of color is also subjective, you and your dentist should evaluate this together.

Moisture and force can cause filling fallout

A few of my tooth-colored bonded fillings recently came out only several days after my dentist put them in. This is the second time they've come out. Is this unusual? At this point I'd almost prefer going to a new dentist.

Composites or tooth-colored fillings can come out for several reasons. Among the most common causes are excessive force on the area during chewing and biting, and moisture levels affecting the filling.

Although composites are used successfully in many areas of the mouth for good functional and aesthetic results, they may fracture or break when used in an area of high stress. For this reason, composites are not often used to restore the biting surfaces of molar or back teeth. Even composite fillings used in areas of wear or decay by the gumline may break off. Although there is no direct biting force in these areas, biting and chewing forces can cause enough of a flexing stress between the filling on the tooth to break the seal between the filling and tooth.

Composite bonding fillings are very sensitive to moisture levels. If there is any moisture contamination during the placement of a filling, either from the mouth or air, the seal between filling and tooth may become weakened. Even after successful placement, the ongoing abrupt changes in moisture from intense sunlight drying out a tooth and from the mouth's wetting the tooth can be enough to cause these fillings to break off.

If a composite filling comes out several times, an alternate restoration should be considered.

Home bleach kits are now believed safe

How safe are home bleaching kits? I'm interested in whitening my teeth but have heard so many conflicting opinions that I'm unsure of what to do.

Short-term studies have indicated that many home bleaching kits used under the supervision of a dentist are safe.

Initially there were concerns by the Food and Drug Administration and the American Dental Association for two reasons. First, many bleaching systems were sold directly to consumers without adequate safety regulations. These kits did not need to meet FDA requirements since they were sold as cosmetic products. Changes have now been made to require more regulation on the sale of such products. Second, long-term studies on those kits that met FDA standards were of concern to some researchers and dentists. Short-term studies have shown minimal impact to the gum tissue. More long-term studies will become available as the use of bleaching systems continue.

Maxillary or upper tray worn on the teeth

Whitener gel

Tooth Whiteners

Whiteners are effective in varying degrees. They are applied to teeth with a plastic customized tray. They bleach the teeth to the desired whiteness.

With many concerns being satisfied, home bleaching is considered generally safe and is recommended by many dentists for patients seeking a whiter smile. To satisfy additional concerns from dental practitioners, several changes have been made to newer bleaching kits. Custom trays are made to prevent extensive leakage of the bleaching solutions on to the surrounding gum tissue. Solutions are made viscous and are able to remain in an isolated area.

Receding gum shows the true color of a crown

I had several caps on my front teeth done several years ago and now notice a graying color at the gumline. Are these decaying, and should they be replaced?

The graying coloration is likely the metal edge of your crown. Decay extensive enough to show a gray color by the gumline would have easily been detected by your dentist.

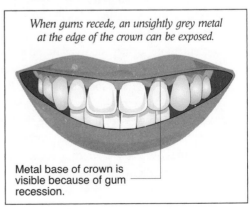

When gums recede, an unsightly grey metal at the edge of the crown can be exposed.

Metal base of crown is visible because of gum recession.

When a crown is first placed, the metal edge is usually below the gumline. However, gum recession or trauma may expose this edge, which will give a gray coloration. Because the amount of porcelain at the gumline is often thin, it can break off in this area, exposing the underlying gray metal color. In such a case, your dentist may be able to bond a white covering to the metal. But even the best techniques fall short of completely masking out the gray.

Should the coloration be aesthetically displeasing, you may want a new crown.

Certain crown designs can help avoid the future possibility of this graying coloration. For example, some porcelain crowns can be made with thicker areas of porcelain by the gumline. Even with gum recession, these will not show the gray color. The disadvantage is the need to remove more tooth structure to compensate for the added thickness of the porcelain.

Other crowns called porcelain jacket crowns are made of porcelain with no gold metal alloy core. Aesthetically these look the most natural, but often are not as strong as other types.

You should consider all the benefits and risks of each crown design with your dentist when choosing a type of crown.

Tooth whitening, a day at the bleach

Does laser bleaching really work?
What are the safest and most effective ways to bleach your teeth?

Laser bleaching is a form of light-activated tooth whitening, and yes it works quite well. What is more important to ask is how safe the procedure is. Most bleaching techniques use different forms and concentrations of peroxide solutions and gels. Dispensing these solutions has traditionally been accompanied by custom trays molded to the teeth. New strips and adhesive plastics which adhere directly to the teeth can be bought as over the counter products in the pharmacy and are also effective. Bleaching methods with gels alone are usually safe. Stronger concentrations of peroxide can sometimes produce gum and tooth sensitivity. In these cases, the products should be discontinued and you should consult with your dentist on other products or methods.

Light activated solutions are more effective for tooth whitening. However, results from studies in 2004 indicate that there may be potential risks of heating teeth. Bleaching done with lasers produce the highest temperature increase. Both argon and CO_2 lasers which are commonly used by dentists produce effects which are conclusively more dramatic. Dentists and patients must be aware that there can be associated risks to the teeth as heat increases are a form of trauma to the structure and nerves of the teeth.

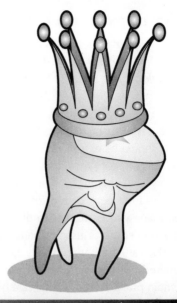

Chapter 7

Crowns and Bridges

Fixed Prosthodontics
- Prostho (prosthesis)
- fixed appliance to restore teeth

Dentists prefer saving teeth to removing them

One of my upper back teeth is decayed down to the gumline. Now to fix it, the dentist wants to cut the gums around the tooth. How will that help? Wouldn't it be easier to have the tooth removed?

As long as a tooth is firmly anchored in bone, it may provide years of use. A large decayed or broken area above the gumline doesn't necessarily mean the tooth should be extracted. However, because there is little area above the gumline left, surgical procedures are needed to expose more tooth area.

"Crown lengthening" is a procedure that involves removing gum and/or bone around the neck or root of a tooth. A crown or other restoration can then be made which attaches to this exposed area.

The procedure is usually completed in one visit and is only slightly painful. The affected area usually heals in two weeks. Then the tooth can be prepared for a crown or other filling.

Certain problems may complicate or prevent your dentist from completing this procedure. If the gums or bone around the remaining roots are too infected, the underlying bone support may be weakened and unable to support a restoration. Also, the risk of recurring infection may further jeopardize the tooth.

Small teeth with short roots present an additional problem since there is less to work with before the procedure and less root support for a completed restoration.

Your dentist weighs these risks and benefits always in favor of retaining your own teeth. Regardless of how little appears to remain, or how extensive the tooth decay, there may be a way to successfully retain and use such a tooth.

Gumline Surgery

When a crack appears on the tooth close to the gumline, the tooth is not necessarily a lost cause. If the gumline can be lowered with minor surgery, the tooth can be crowned and last for years to come.

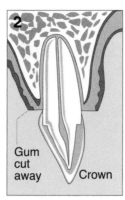

The gumline is cut away and tooth is ground down to allow for crown placement.

After gums heal, the crown is placed over area of crack.

Some fractures can be tough to repair

A piece of my back tooth broke off after biting down on a bone. My dentist recommended crowning the whole tooth but told me that there was a risk that the tooth may not be restorable. What would prevent him from repairing my tooth?

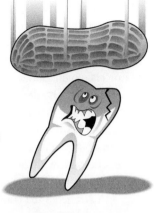

Tooth fractures are common. They can vary from a minor chip to a complete fracture of tooth and roots.

The degree of the fracture depends on the resistance of the tooth, the angle of contact and hardness of the material causing the fracture.

Fractures are more common in teeth already compromised with existing fillings. Tooth surfaces surrounding a large filling on the biting area of back teeth are particularly prone to fracture. For this reason, your dentist may recommend replacing large silver or composite fillings with cast gold or porcelain coverings which may better protect the tooth from fracturing.

The location and extent of a fracture may determine the likelihood of success in repairing the area. For example, if a molar fractures below the gumline near or below the level of bone supporting the tooth, your dentist may have difficulty or be unable to adequately restore the area.

It is important to prevent fractures by locating teeth that are prone to such incidents and protecting them with sufficient restorations. Habits like chewing ice, hard candy or popcorn can also cause fractures in an otherwise healthy and strong tooth.

A crown of gold may mean more stability

My dentist tells me that he cannot make a porcelain crown on my back tooth because it's too short. "Gold is better," he says. Can you tell me about a possible compromise if I don't like the way gold looks?

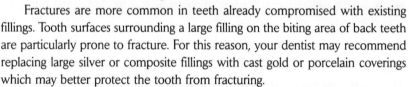

Many factors determine the type of filling used to restore a tooth. Most crowns can be widely classified into three categories: porcelain, metal or a combination of the two.

Crowns made of metal, usually a gold alloy, are preferred in many cases. Less tooth structure needs to be removed, and the final crown wears evenly against an opposing natural tooth. Porcelain crowns or a combination of metal and porcelain require more tooth structure to be removed. Also, if there is a porcelain biting surface, an opposing natural tooth can begin to wear faster since porcelain is a harder material.

A tooth that is "short" implies that the portion of the tooth above the gumline is smaller than normal. Since more of the tooth needs to be removed to make a porcelain crown with a metal core, very little above the gum would be left. A crown placed on such a foundation has difficulty staying in. If one makes a gold or metal crown, less tooth needs to be removed.

If aesthetics still concern you, inform your dentist. You should only proceed on work that has aesthetic priorities after discussing the functional risks with your dentist.

Porcelain restoration improves aesthetics

A section of the porcelain covering on one tooth chipped off.
The tooth doesn't bother me, other than leaving a rough surface.
Can this just be left missing, without replacing the cap?

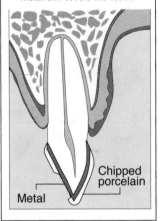

Porcelain Chipping

Porcelain crowns that chip don't usually need immediate attention because underlying metal still covers the tooth.

Chipped porcelain

Metal

One common type of crown or cap is made of porcelain with an underlying metal shell.

After years of wear, sections of the porcelain may fracture and break away, leaving portions of the metal shell exposed. When this occurs, there is usually no harm done to the tooth underneath. The metal protects the tooth.

Immediate attention is usually not required unless a sharp or rough edge cuts or aggravates surrounding areas like the cheek and tongue. However, you should see your dentist to evaluate any need to eventually replace the restoration.

If the porcelain chips or breaks away either on the biting surface or between neighboring teeth, the crown often needs to be replaced. If the fracture occurs in other areas where aesthetics are more of a concern, a patient may sometimes choose to have the remaining surface smoothed and/or contoured.

Slow drilling is needed for some dental work

My dentist used a slow-speed drill in the final stages of cleaning out the decay in a tooth. It felt rather uncomfortable; why are these used?

When a tooth has decay near or close to the pulp or central nerve of your tooth, your dentist uses caution when removing the infection. Slower-speed drills and hand-instruments are less traumatic to the nerve.

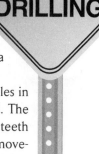

However, you often feel a vibration or scraping sensation which you may perceive as being more traumatic to the tooth.

Because the high-speed drill goes so fast, a patient is often unable to perceive the amount or depth of the tooth structure being removed. High-speed drills also create considerable heat, which is why they are cooled by a stream of water as they function.

Slow-speed drills are also used for preparing holes in designated areas that will have posts or pins placed. The slow speed is useful for contouring and smoothing teeth and fillings. Because less heat is generated by their movement, such drills are used in more delicate functions that require slower removal of material with less trauma.

Determining location of crown margins

The last time I had a crown done, I could see the edge by the gumline. I prefer that the edges do not show. My dentist, however, told me it is healthier for the gum tissue just the way it is and that edges extending below the gumline often irritate the tissue. Is that true? If so, why aren't all crowns made that way?

The location of edges or margins of a crown are determined by many factors. Among them are gum tissue considerations, the degree and location of decay, oral hygiene, reshaping of the tooth contours and aesthetics. With all conditions ideal, margins placed above the gumline are the location of choice. They are easier to clean and less likely to irritate the surrounding gums.

Crown Margin

Crown margins that are above the gumline allow the tooth to be better taken care of, but aesthetically the tooth looks better with the margin below the gumline

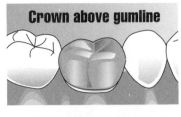
Crown above gumline

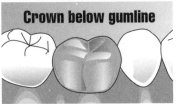
Crown below gumline

In many instances, however, margins are placed below the gumline. Porcelain crowns made for front teeth usually are designed with no margins showing. If there is an area of decay extending below the gumline, regardless of where the tooth is located, the margin of the crown must contain and cover that area. Extra hygiene care is needed for the crown since decay-causing bacteria can more readily collect around margin areas, below the gumline. These crowns may be more likely to develop recession and periodontal disease at a later time.

Crowns won't always last for a lifetime

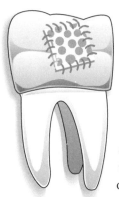

Why do some crowns need to be patched? One of my crowns has only been in for a few years and already my dentist tells me there is an area of possible decay.

With ideal conditions, construction, and good oral hygiene, a crown can last a lifetime. More commonly, one of those variables is at fault. In such cases, crowns or caps can develop areas that require patching or repair. Areas between the crown and tooth can break down from decay, fractures or wear from heavy chewing forces.

The most common source of breakdown or need for repair arises from decay that occurs at the margin between the metal or porcelain crown and the tooth. With diligent oral hygiene, such problems can be prevented. Fractures can occur at the gumline or any area where there is tooth or root structure not covered by the crown.

Wear commonly occurs on the biting surface. Over time, metal wears away as do the biting surfaces of teeth. This wear can perforate the metal casting and create a small opening. If not repaired or patched, this small opening can eventually cause a small hole. If left untreated, the cement seal between the crown and tooth will eventually break.

Retraction cord helps crowns fit snugly

There's some type of string that the dentist packs around your gums before taking a mold for a new crown. What is it and what does it do?

After the tooth has been drilled and prepared for a new crown, a string-like material called retraction cord is placed around the edges by the gumline. The edges, or margins must form a tight seal with the new crown for it to be successful long-term.

Retraction cord acts to push away gum tissue from these margin areas. Then when the mold is taken, and the cord is removed, material can accurately record the margins. If gum tissue is inflamed or irritated, other steps must be taken to help control the tissue. Anticoagulants may be used to stop bleeding. Electrosurgery or laser surgery also can help control tissue that would otherwise interfere with recording an accurate mold. After these steps are taken, the retraction cord can be placed to control remaining gum tissue around the prepared area.

Retraction Cord

Before an impression or mold is taken of a tooth, cord is used to pull the tissue away. This allows a more accurate mold of the gumline area.

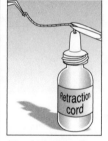
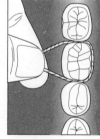

A two inch piece of retraction cord is cut.

A loop is formed around the tooth and pulled tight.

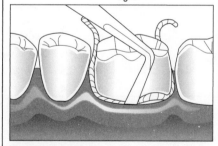

The retraction cord is pushed slightly under the gingiva.

To help your dentist, meticulous oral hygiene care can help reduce any gum inflammation and swelling. This will help alleviate the need for additional steps. Often tissue removal and control of bleeding are needed for people with gum disease as a result of poor oral hygiene.

Getting a crown mold may be a royal pain

The last time a crown was made for one of my lower teeth, my dentist had to take three molds of the same area. He said it was a difficult case. My previous dentist needed to take only one mold whenever a crown was made. What determines a hard case?

Several factors determine the difficulty in taking a mold. They can be broadly described as characteristics of the patient and of the tooth that requires the crown. Patients who tend to gag more easily, swallow frequently, or who are unable to open their mouths widely for long periods, or who have small mouths, all present difficulty. Any movement by the patient during the impression or mold-taking process must be controlled. Until impression materials harden they are prone to distortion. In general, lower teeth present more problems because of the reactions of the tongue.

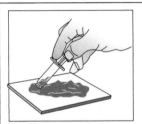

Impression material is mixed on a board and is loaded into a syringe.

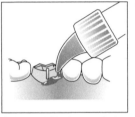

The material is then applied to the crowning area called the sulcus.

The patient's cooperation has a lot to do with how successful a crown mold will be. Here is how a mold is taken for a crown:

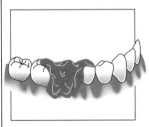

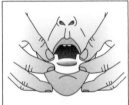

A tray is inserted on top of the impression material and is removed when the mold is set.

The condition, position and shape of the teeth to be recorded can affect the outcome of an impression. Teeth badly broken and difficult to restore are usually hard to record with molds. Problems such as excessive bleeding associated with gum irritation and inflammation create additional problems. Some teeth are in awkward positions or have odd shapes and are either at an unusual angle or close to other structures of the mouth, making the mold-taking process more difficult.

A Post strengthens a tooth but could still fracture

How does a post, put in a tooth, break?

A metal post is often placed in a tooth which is badly broken down or requires additional support to withstand chewing force. The posts are of varying widths and lengths of materials such as stainless steel, titanium and gold. They are cemented into one or more of the empty nerve canals of root-canal-treated teeth. Although they can help strengthen the tooth, they, like healthy teeth, are susceptible to fracture.

If the root cracks or is fractured when the post breaks, the remaining root may need to be removed. When a post breaks at or above the gumline the tooth can usually

Posts and Pins

Posts can strengthen teeth that have had root canals, but these posts or pins can break. Here is how they are made:

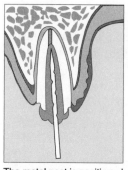
The metal post is positioned into the acrylic mold.

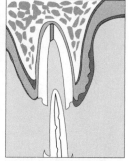
The mold is removed and shaped into a replacement.

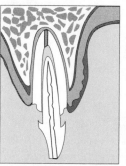
The replacement, with post included, is cemented back in tooth base.

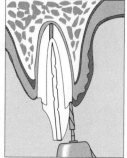
The replacement is then shaped and finished with drill.

be restored. The remaining fractured post can often not be replaced by a new post as the opening is sealed by the old broken post. Posts are permanently cemented into the nerve canals, making their removal nearly impossible and always risky.

To restore the tooth, the dentist may have to find alternative ways besides using a post. If the tooth has many roots, like back molar teeth, a smaller post can possibly be anchored in one of the remaining nerve cells. But if the tooth has no other areas for additional posts, pins and other weaker build-up materials are used; these will often not be as strong as the original post and therefore may break. They may, however, provide the only option for restoring the tooth.

Temporaries keep teeth in position

My temporary has a metallic taste and seems to trap food more easily. Isn't there something better that dentists can use while the final cap is being made?

Temporary crowns protect teeth that have been prepared for permanent restorations. In addition, temporaries help maintain the tooth position and biting relationship to the surrounding teeth.

There are a wide variety of materials and cements that can be used for temporary fillings. Temporary crowns, however, are usually made from metal or acrylic. Front teeth are commonly made from tooth-colored acrylic, while back teeth are often covered with a molded metal cap that restores the repaired tooth to its normal size and shape.

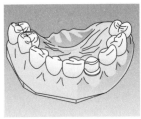

A plaster cast is taken of the mouth and the prepared tooth.

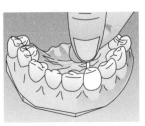

The temporary is molded to fit the plaster cast and cemented into place in the mouth.

Temporaries are worn for usually a week or two although they can be made to last longer. They are held onto the tooth by a temporary cement so that they will not easily dislodge while eating.

Temporaries

Temporaries are a step taken between the cleaning of a decaying tooth and the placement of a crown. Here are some of the steps taken:

Because the anatomy and shape of teeth are so difficult to reproduce in a final crown, a well-made temporary can be a long, involved process. Time and expense do not always permit your dentist to make an ideal temporary. So there may be problems associated with them. A metallic taste may be caused by contact with a dissimilar metal used in other fillings around the temporary. If you have a tendency to trap more food between your teeth, the temporary tooth contour may vary slightly from ideal, creating a space where food can get caught. Occasionally, surrounding gums may get inflamed if the edge of a temporary pushes on or against an area by the gumline. Your dentist will want to avoid such instances. Let him or her know of any discomfort, as it may be easily adjusted or changed. A good temporary often helps ensure an easy and well-adjusted fit for a permanent crown.

Cement creates a lasting bond between tooth, cap

One of my crowns came off recently,
and my dentist put it back in with some special cement.
Aren't all caps glued in with the same type of cement?

There are many types of cements used in dentistry. Some are specific for a single purpose while others can be used for many procedures. Two dentists may use different cements for the same purpose. Even routine procedures like cementing crowns are done with different types of cements.

Each cement has its advantages and disadvantages. Some form a stronger bond to the tooth surface while others prevent decay from spreading underneath a crown. Newer types of cements bond directly to metal, making a seal stronger to a metallic surface.

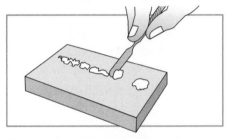

Cement powder is mixed with a liquid agent to create the applicable cement solution.

Cementing the Deal

There are different types of cement
for different dental jobs. Here are
how some cements are applied:

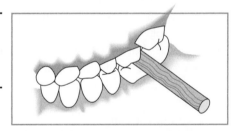

After the crown is applied with the cement, the patient is asked to bite on a piece of cotton, wood or plastic to press the crown down firmly around its tooth core.

If your dislodged crown fits precisely into place, one of several standard cements is used. If there are holes or openings in or around the crown, then a special cement may be needed. Many standard cements will dissolve away when exposed. Thus cementing a crown with an opening requires a cement that will fill this area and not dissolve.

Ideally any crown with such an opening should be re-made to fit the prepared area in the tooth. However, some of the newer cements offer a less costly, but adequate, alternative to remaking a crown.

Crowning touch will ease biting problems

My husband recently had a crown put in.
He felt okay for a while but now says that it hits first when he bites.
Will this sensation pass or should the crown be adjusted?

When a crown or filling is made, the biting surface is carved or formed to match the original tooth. The surface has a complex array of grooves and bumps which contact specific areas of opposing teeth when you bite and chew. Slight alterations in the height and position of these bumps and grooves can alter the way your teeth meet when you bite. These alterations can have a dramatic effect on both your ability to chew effectively and the overall health of restored teeth.

If one of the bumps is too high or a groove is not deep enough to accommodate the bump of an opposing tooth when you bite together, the tooth "hits first." Minor adjustments allow teeth to contact more evenly. When the crown is first placed, your dentist errs on the side of not relieving enough of this biting surface since he can always remove material. However, if your dentist takes away too much of the biting surface, the tooth may not function ideally when you chew. A tooth may feel comfortable but can cause damage that shows up later as discomfort in nearby teeth or in the jaw joint.

Since your husband feels the tooth contacting first, he should see the dentist for an additional adjustment. Often the tooth or jaw is numb at the time it is cemented, so it may be difficult to sense high areas. Other factors influence tooth contact, including posture, head position and your individual pattern of chewing.

Research shows that a person can distinguish a high surface on a tooth that varies by as little as 1/25,000 of an inch. The quality of refining this surface to match your original bite is thus challenging even for the most experienced dentist.

Crown Finishing

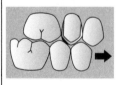

A crown that has a "bump" or protrusive prematurity can push teeth and cause them to shift positions.

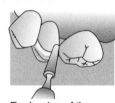

Reshaping of the crown can be done with burnishing tools and polystone rotating tools.

Defective crown may hide an infection

My crown on my back tooth has a small hole on top.
The dentist told me it should be removed and replaced with a
new one. Can't the small hole just be filled?

Bacteria can enter any small hole or defect in a crown. If the area goes undetected for several months, the decay may extend deep into the underlying tooth. The tooth beneath the crown must be uncovered to remove deep or extensive decay.

If caught early, decay may be repaired without removing the crown. During regular examination, crown defects can sometimes be detected. However, infection around crowns is not always painful and can go unnoticed for months. Even x-rays may miss such areas.

Indicators of defects around crowns include sensitivity to hot and cold foods, fraying of floss when placed between the teeth and areas around teeth that more readily trap food.

Regular checkups and alerting your dentist of symptoms may save both healthy tooth structure under crowns and the cost of replacing crowns.

Caps provide a needed anchor for dentures

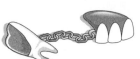

As part of getting my mouth ready for a partial den-
ture, our family dentist wants to put caps on several
of my teeth. Are these caps necessary?

Existing teeth often need to be crowned or capped in order to achieve a well-fitting denture. New crowns can be custom made with slots or depressions in one or more of their surfaces that later will attach to the partial denture. Such fittings prevent the denture from moving while you talk and eat.

Using your natural teeth or teeth with existing fillings may not be adequate for several reasons. Large silver fillings, for example, may fracture and break from the stresses of fittings that link a partial denture to your tooth.

Teeth with no fillings also may need to be crowned. They may be angled in a direction that varies from their ideal position. A denture may be difficult to fit around such malpositioned teeth. By crowning these teeth, one can achieve a more ideal angle and position.

There are many factors that determine the success of your denture. Crowning ensures a proper fit and a reliable tooth base for the denture.

Dentist should bridge gaps in crown work

My gums have been irritated for several months around the back part of my bridgework. My dentist tells me that there is an "open margin" causing the irritation and that he may have to replace the bridge. What causes this and are there any easier ways to repair it?

An open margin describes an opening between the free edge of a crown and the tooth it covers. Normally, these areas are tightly sealed, but over time, the supporting tooth which a crown covers can become decayed or eroded.

Causes of an open margin include plaque accumulation leading to decay, erosion from acidic juices or regurgitation of stomach acids, as in the case of bulimics and abnormal stresses of chewing and biting. Searching for these areas is one of many parts of a routine examination.

Gap in Bridgework

An open margin can lead to decay or other complications. This should be filled by your dentist, or in more severe cases, the bridge might have to be replaced.

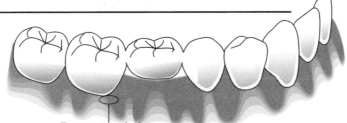

**Decay area below
gumline margin of crown**

There are some signs and symptoms which may indicate an open margin. Two such signs are when a tooth becomes more temperature sensitive or begins to fray the floss when you are cleaning it. However, many times there are no indications, and detection by your dentist or hygienist can be difficult. Once detected, an open margin can be repaired by cleaning out the open space and closing it with a filling.

If the opening is too large or if the decay cannot be adequately removed, the crown or bridge may need to be removed. Decay in and around an open margin can also cause structural damage to the underlying tooth and may affect the support of bridgework, sometimes causing a fracture or break in either the tooth or bridgework.

Bridgework depends on basic engineering

When restoring my upper teeth with a bridge, the dentist wants to use three of my healthy teeth to hold the bridge. Why can't he just use two since he has to drill an otherwise perfectly healthy tooth?

When designing bridgework, your dentist considers a law of physical engineering called "Ante's law." Basically, the law helps determine the minimum amount of tooth support needed to restore a given area where teeth are missing. So, for example, if you were missing only one back tooth, perhaps only two healthy teeth would be needed to hold and support a bridge. However, if you were missing two teeth next to each other, you might require three supporting teeth.

To appreciate the law, imagine that for every tooth lost, the remaining teeth must compensate for the work of that single tooth. The more missing teeth, the greater the stress on the surrounding teeth.

The health of the teeth used as supports is also an important factor. Even in cases where one tooth is missing, additional supports may be needed if these surrounding teeth have periodontal disease or bone loss around them. In more severe cases, fixed bridgework may not even be an option to restore an area as the supporting teeth cannot hold up to the stresses of biting and chewing.

Bridge Support

The support for bridge work may be determined by the amount of teeth missing.

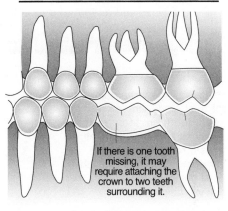

If there is one tooth missing, it may require attaching the crown to two teeth surrounding it.

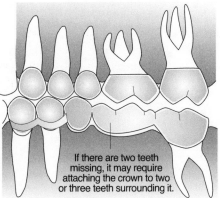

If there are two teeth missing, it may require attaching the crown to two or three teeth surrounding it.

A Bridge clears the gumline for sanitary reasons

When my dentist put in a bridge on my lower teeth, I noticed that the artificial tooth rested high above the gumline. How come it doesn't rest directly on the gums?

Artificial teeth on a bridge are called pontics. These have no underlying roots or attachments to the jaw as do the bridge ends, which are usually cemented over prepared teeth. Although they may be constructed in many different ways, there are two broad categories of pontics. Those that touch the gumline are referred to as ridge lap. Pontics that rest above the gumline are called sanitary. In general, sanitary pontics are used more often when making lower bridges while ridgelap pontics are common in bridges restoring upper teeth.

Sanitary pontics don't look as natural because only the biting surface and about one-third of the tooth body is present. However, they are easier to keep clean and seldom trap or lodge food particles. Ridgelap pontics have an aesthetic advantage.

Bridge Over Troubled Gumline

Bridgework creates a substitute for a missing tooth in order to keep teeth in their proper positions and to support biting pressures. The bridge is sometimes placed in a way that does not touch the gumline for hygiene purposes.

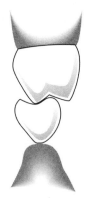

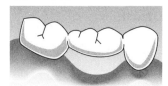

This shows a ridge lap pontic touching the gumline.

When well made, an artificial tooth is more difficult to distinguish from a real one. But because artificial teeth touch the gumline, small food particles can wedge in between the gum and teeth. Plaque and tartar are more likely to build up on the underlying surface, which is more difficult to keep clean.

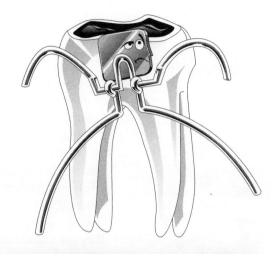

Chapter 8

Braces and Moving Teeth

Orthodontics
- Ortho (straighten or correct)

Misalignment of jaw needs early diagnosis

According to our dentist, our son has a crossbite on one side of his jaw. Can you explain what exactly that is? How can it be treated, and what happens if it's just left alone?

Crossbites

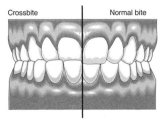

Crossbite | Normal bite

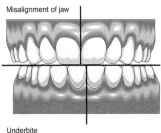

Misalignment of jaw

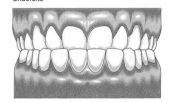

Underbite

Upper teeth normally overlap lower teeth when you bite. If the biting surfaces of your lower teeth are clearly visible or overlap the upper teeth when the jaw is closed, a crossbite is present.

Proper alignment of your teeth is important for several reasons. First, chewing efficiency increases. Second, jaw mobility and muscle activity is balanced and unhindered. Third, excessive and abnormal tooth wear can be avoided more easily.

Crossbites can appear in any part of the jaw. They are usually defined at an early age. They may result from teeth being out of position or from discrepancies in jaw bone development.

Treatment includes orthodontics and oral surgery depending on the degree of discrepancy. If not treated, complications such as tooth abrasion, jaw joint problems and chewing and speaking difficulties may result. Early diagnosis and treatment is beneficial as developing bone can be shaped and guided with appliances. Such early intervention may prevent surgery that would be necessary if initial treatment were delayed until adulthood.

Braces early on may help keep jaw in line

Our seven-year-old son has a severe bite problem.
When I took him to our dentist, it was suggested that he see
an orthodontist. Is it too early?
All of the kids I see wearing braces are teens.

In the past, braces were traditionally placed on teenagers' teeth to correct poorly formed bites. The earliest age to visit the orthodontist used to be 12 years. Now, however, there are situations when braces and other appliances can be useful at a much younger age.

If one starts at an early age, many features of development and growth can work with the dentist to help correct a problem. Sometimes, the size of the jaw does not match the amount of space needed to allow correct positioning of teeth. Correcting these variables at an early age is often easier than waiting until development is more complete. For example, if jaw size is not adequate to accommodate future adult teeth, an appliance can be made to expand the jaw. As long as this expansion occurs during development, the jaw can easily be molded.

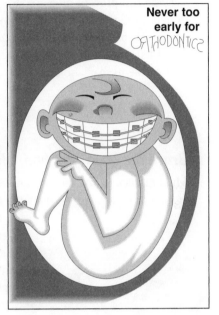

Never too early for ORTHODONTICS

Current practice concentrates on predicting the future outcome of the correct position of teeth in the jaw. Even children under age five may benefit from some type of orthodontic appliance. Your dentist should recognize that the possibility of orthodontics at this early age may help dental development in later years.

Thumb-sucking can cause "open bite"

Our family dentist is referring our ten-year-old son to an orthodontist for an "open bite". What causes this and how is it treated? Is there anything we could have done as parents to prevent this from happening?

An "open bite" describes a condition where there is an open space between the biting surfaces of upper and lower teeth when the jaws are closed. Although the condition occurs most often with front teeth, any area of the jaw can be affected.

Most cases of an open bite result from thumb sucking and tongue thrusting habits. Other developmental factors such as prolonged retention of baby teeth and abnormal eruption of permanent teeth can cause open bites. In these cases, teeth normally having flexibility in their attachment to the jaw bone are fused to the bone.

Treatment of open bites are as varied as the causes. As long as oral habits such as thumb-sucking are stopped by age six, open bites can usually be avoided in the front teeth. If habits persist past this age, orthodontic appliances are suggested to prevent on-going pressure on the teeth. Other muscle and jaw exercises are recommended for other situations. Treatment should begin at a young age, before ten years, if problems are detected early.

If left untreated, chewing food can become more difficult. Muscle and joint problems may also arise.

Brace for good and bad when choosing ceramics

My daughter wants ceramic braces and fillings on her teeth instead of metal ones. What's the difference?

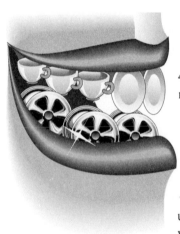

Ceramic braces and fillings match the color of the teeth, so they're cosmetically superior. Ceramic fillings also are superior to many filling materials. They cost more, as much as 400 percent more for fillings and 30 percent more for braces.

Several other factors may influence your choice for ceramic braces and fillings.

Ceramic braces can cause tooth wear for people with a deep overbite. Ceramic braces attached to the outer surface of lower front teeth can contact the inside surfaces of your upper front teeth. If you have such a problem, your orthodontist will substitute plastic brackets on your lower front teeth.

People considering porcelain fillings should be more concerned with tooth wear. If the porcelain contacts a natural tooth surface while chewing, it will slowly erode the tooth's enamel surface. To avoid such wear, gold fillings may be a wiser choice. Tooth-colored cast composite fillings also avoid tooth wear but are not as durable as gold.

Ceramic braces may be an appropriate choice for your daughter, but you may want to consider the durability and wear of gold when deciding between ceramic and gold fillings.

Orthodontics best for aligning teeth

*My lower front teeth are out of alignment,
and they've been bothering me. Is there an easy,
inexpensive way to correct them without doing caps?*

Tooth alignment problems are best corrected with orthodontics. In most cases, moving teeth with brackets and wires is sufficient and easy, although it may not be inexpensive. Depending upon the degree and difficulty of moving the teeth, orthodontic treatment may take months to a couple of years to properly finish. After completion, a retainer, either removable or fixed to the teeth, is placed to prevent teeth moving back to their original positions.

Composite tooth-colored bonding materials or porcelain coverings called laminates also may be used to aesthetically correct poorly aligned teeth. These may be less costly and be completed in two weeks or less. However, only in cases where alignment problems are slight and are not involved in other bite problems should this option be explored. In many instances, these restorations can give beautiful and natural-looking results.

Your dentist will review options related to your case as all have unique differences and factors that may affect the outcome.

Metal bands on braces can cover up decay

Before braces are put on my teeth, my family dentist wants to do some fillings. He suggests that I have crowns done after the braces come off. Why are some fillings done before and some after braces? Are there any advantages to having all the work done before the braces are put on?

Before braces are placed, your dentist should complete a thorough examination. Any decayed or broken-down teeth should be restored before braces are attached. If decayed areas are not restored at this time, serious consequences may result.

Metal bands are commonly placed around back molar teeth. These bands may cover decayed areas for several years during orthodontic treatment. Diagnostic instruments and x-rays cannot detect these areas, so decay may progress and be extensive once the bands are removed. Likewise, other areas of decay are difficult to repair while braces are on the teeth.

Some restorative work such as certain crowns or cast fillings can be completed after orthodontic treatment. In this way, spaces created or not closed during orthodontic treatment can be corrected at the same time as the restorative work is being completed.

Brace yourself: Oral hygiene prevents spots

Our daughter has white spots on her teeth since her braces were taken off. Can anything be done to correct the spots? Also, is there anything that can prevent this?

White spots can be present on teeth after orthodontic treatment. They are related directly to oral hygiene practices during the time the braces are worn. Patients with poor brushing and flossing habits are more likely to develop these spots. White spots have a greater chance of forming the longer braces remain on teeth, particularly when treatment extends beyond two years.

There are some preventive measures which will decrease the possibility of white spots forming. Rinses of sodium fluoride after brushing with a fluoride toothpaste have been shown to decrease the likelihood of these spots forming. Your orthodontist or general dentist usually will suggest a method of hygiene to adequately prevent problems such as white spots from forming.

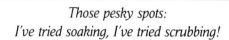

Those pesky spots:
I've tried soaking, I've tried scrubbing!

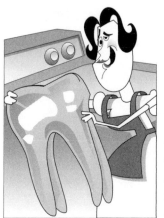

Braces often make the chore of cleaning teeth more difficult. Extra care is needed to remove food debris and plaque. More frequent cleanings at your general dentist's office may be indicated during the time your child wears braces.

Once the spots have formed, it may be difficult to reverse the process. There are some techniques, which involve applying solutions to the teeth, that can reverse mild forms of white spots. However, in more severe cases, bonded fillings or porcelain coverings may be the best choice.

Pressure can correct poor teeth alignment

Our eight-year-old daughter has crowded upper teeth.
Her dentist suggested she wear a device that would increase her jaw
size. How does this work? Are there other solutions?

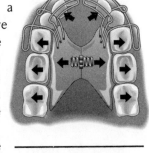

Your dentist has probably recommended a palatal-expansion appliance. During the formative years, bones are still developing and are responsive to pushing and pulling. It is therefore possible to use pressure to mold the bones of your daughter's jaw. Once an ideal shape or size is determined, an appliance designed by your dentist will provide the desired result.

Expansion devices are either attached to the teeth with metal rings that fit over the teeth or with removable plastic plates worn in the mouth. Each has a spring-loaded wire or expandable screw that can be adjusted to put pressure on an area of bone.

Crowded teeth can be corrected with a palatal-expansion appliance by your orthodontist. Pressure to expand the jaw in formative years can correct misaligned teeth.

These instruments are made for the upper or lower jaw and must be adjusted periodically. They often need to be worn several years.

Crowded teeth may be corrected through other methods. If a patient has enough jaw space, but the teeth are not aligned properly, moving them with braces may correct the problem.

Lost retainer must be replaced quickly

Our daughter recently lost her retainer.
She's been wearing it for about a year.
Do we need to get another one made?
What happens if another one is not worn?

Retainers are commonly used to stabilize teeth after orthodontic treatment. They are usually made of a clear acrylic plastic and wire, which holds the teeth in their desired position. As a general rule, retainers should be worn for the same length of time as braces were worn. Adults usually need to wear them for longer periods.

Movement of teeth during the time braces are worn puts a stress on the ligaments that hold the root of the tooth to the surrounding bone. After such forces are removed, some teeth want to move back to their original position, thus relieving the tension on the ligaments. Retainers hold the teeth during a period when the ligaments and bone can adapt to a tooth's new position.

Should you lose or misplace a retainer, a replacement needs to be made promptly. Without a retainer, teeth can begin to move within hours. Should several months pass before a new retainer is made, teeth may drift permanently out of position. The new retainer can only prevent such teeth from moving further, but in many cases cannot guide the tooth back to its original position.

Space for teeth is expanded four ways

Our son's teeth seem to be crowding together.
The orthodontist agrees that treatment is needed.
How can space be provided without removing a lot of teeth?

There are four methods to create space for crowded teeth. Depending on factors such as age, facial profile, jaw development and amount of space needed, one or more of these methods may be used.

Expansion of the jaw seems like a useful and obvious means to gain needed space. However, only a limited amount of space can be achieved and is best done during normal growth periods. In general, the back areas of the jaw are the most responsive to expansion techniques. Usually an appliance is worn that puts pressure on the bone to expand outward.

One of the most common methods to gain space is to reduce the number of teeth. In many cases, the extraction of teeth allows sufficient space for remaining teeth to be guided into a proper alignment. In some cases, where only a limited amount of space is needed, teeth can be filed so that the width is more narrow. A procedure called stripping removes some of the outer enamel so that the overall width of a tooth is reduced.

The last two categories utilize the same principle in different ways. Distilizing refers to the method of pushing posterior teeth back further, allowing more room for crowded teeth in the front. Advancing, on the other hand, is a method for pushing front teeth further forward, allowing for more room in crowded back areas.

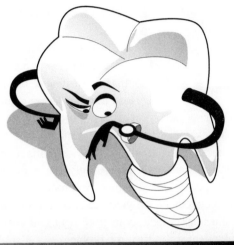

Chapter 9

Emergency Care

Aspirin may not chase toothache away

My father told me to put some aspirin next to my tooth when it gets sore. The next time I tried it, some of the pain went away, but it still hurt. What's the best way to treat a toothache?

The best way to treat a toothache is to see a dentist. There are many problems and sources that lead to a toothache. Treating or taking medications on your own can likely lead to more severe complications.

Placing aspirin on or near a tooth that aches is common. However, it is a classic example of a home remedy that will lead to further problems. Chemicals in the aspirin kill the tissue surface of your gums and cheek. A white layer forms and then eventually sheds, exposing an underlying painful lesion. This exposed area can then be prone to infection. Aspirin should never be placed directly on the gums, cheeks or lips for a prolonged time. Taking aspirin or other pain medications is all right and even recommended for tooth pain until a dentist can treat the problem.

There are many agents sold to cure a toothache. Many are gels or ointments that act as an anesthetic to numb an area. Although these may work for some tooth and gum pain, they often do not manage many problems associated with a toothache.

Beware of advertisers who may simplify the treatment of tooth pain or claim that there is one agent that provides relief.

Home remedies help for short-term relief

Are there any tips you can give for treating a toothache should one happen on a sailing trip we plan to take?

Several home remedies may help a toothache when you're not able to get professional help. For chipped or broken teeth, plug or cover the fractured area to avoid sharp edges of the tooth from cutting your tongue, lips or cheeks. Sugarless gum or orthodontic wax, available at the pharmacy or from your dentist, are both useful.

Painful or swollen gums may be relieved by rinsing with a teaspoon of table or sea salt in a cup of warm water. You may also use hydrogen peroxide diluted in half with water. Anesthetic gels may provide some temporary relief but usually require frequent application.

If a crown or bridge should come off, try to gently dry off the teeth and reattach them using either orthodontic wax or denture adhesive.

With all toothaches, avoid foods that are difficult to chew and extreme changes in liquid and food temperatures. Avoid foods with small seeds.

If you have problems with recurring dental infections, you may want to ask your dentist for specific emergency treatments.

Sometimes your dentist will advise you to take an antibiotic and pain medication with you in case of an emergency. Only take antibiotics and other prescription drugs with specific instructions from your dentist. Indiscriminate use of such medications may complicate and intensify problems.

Even with temporary relief and the best of home care, you should see a dentist immediately for any tooth or gum ache. Delaying treatment may likely result in a more costly and painful problem.

Swollen taste buds are no cause for alarm

One of the taste buds on my tongue is swollen. How long will this burning sensation last, and what should I do to treat it?

Irritation to the various papillae, or taste buds, can cause a swelling and burning sensation of the tongue. Identifying the factor causing the irritation, as well as the location of the affected taste bud, is the first step toward remedying your discomfort.

There are three broad categories of papillae on the tongue. On the back and sides of the tongue closer to your throat are the foliate papillae. These enlarge when irritated and infected. Irritation in this area commonly arises from a fractured tooth edge rubbing against the tongue.

The circumvallate papillae also are located in the back of the exposed tongue surface and are arranged in a V-shaped pattern. Because of their larger size, irritation and enlargement of these areas may cause unnecessary alarm. Along the front surface of the tongue are the fungiform papillae which are concentrated at the tip. Smoking, drinking alcohol and eating hot, spicy foods can cause these papillae to enlarge.

Once a causative factor is found and treated, the irritated papillae will return to normal within a couple of weeks. If the swelling or burning sensation persists, you should see your dentist for a follow-up examination to find and eliminate any additional sources of irritation. In most cases, the size and sensation of the affected taste bud will quickly return to normal.

Air pockets are suspect in pressure pains

I'm an underwater diver and have noticed that on my deep dives, one of my teeth starts throbbing. I recently had a filling in the same tooth. Why does this tooth still bother me?

My first question to you is "does the tooth hurt any other time?" Assuming your answer is no, the pain is probably related to the process of placing the filling in the tooth.

While fillings are being placed or cemented, air pockets may develop either in the filling material or in the cement used. These pockets respond to changes in atmospheric pressure, giving the symptoms you describe. Pressure changes affect your body depending on the depth of your dives, while the trapped air pocket in your filling remains at the same pressure. This pressure difference is the source of your throbbing sensation.

Divers and pilots have this type of pain more often because they undergo dramatic pressure changes in their environment.

What can be done to get rid of this pain? Notify your dentist of the symptoms. He will probably want to replace the filling, attempting to get rid of any air pockets.

Lost tooth need not become a statistic

Our son lost a tooth in a surfing accident.
He came home with the tooth wrapped in
a tissue, and I took him to our family dentist
in hopes of saving it.
Are there better ways to care for a
tooth that's been lost in an accident?

About five million teeth are lost each
year due to accidents, fights and athletics.
Reimplanting the tooth is successful more than 90 percent of the time if you
reach the dentist within 30 minutes.

The American Dental Association and the American Academy of Pediatric
Dentistry recommend placing the tooth in a container of cold whole milk or
saline solution, available in any drug store or pharmacy, to keep outer cells alive.
The cells determine how well the tooth will re-attach to the jaw bone. Wrapping
the tooth in tissue or gauze is not recommended because it causes the cells to
dry out. Putting the tooth on ice is also damaging. Likewise the tooth should not
be rinsed to remove dirt and debris.

Recently, Dr. Paul Krasner, an endodontist (root canal specialist) developed
a prepackaged container with a tooth preserving solution that keeps a tooth
alive for 12 hours. Often an accident will cause more severe body injuries than
those to the teeth. Krasner's system allows a physician to care for trauma
wounds before calling in a dentist.

Foreign objects in food are hazardous

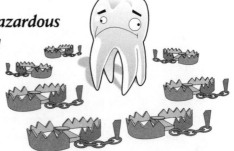

There was a piece of glass in my food
that caused some bleeding in my
mouth, but otherwise I feel okay.
Nothing hurts except a slight
burning sensation on my gums.
Can anything else develop?

Foreign objects in food items can cause a wide variety of problems in the
mouth. Injuries include tooth fracture, lip and gum lacerations, trauma to the
tongue, cheek, palate or throat irritation. Foreign objects found in food range
from glass fragments to plastic and metal objects, stones, shells, bones and wood

splinters. They are most commonly found in candy, baked goods, vegetables and soft drinks.

Because of the variety of objects and the potential damage to various parts of the mouth, you should always have your dentist check your mouth for any additional fragments or damage to structures in the mouth that you may be unable to detect. For example, small sharp objects such as glass or metal fragments can pierce or lodge in soft tissue, which can later be a site for infection. Larger, more blunt objects like stones or pits may fracture or break a tooth or dental filling that is not noticeably painful. Sometimes, resulting damage such as a fracture may not show up for months after the incident. Detecting potential problems can avoid further injury and complications that may result in pain and additional expense to treat.

Fracture requires a wait to determine treatment

*I fell in a bicycle accident, and my dentist
told me I fractured the root of my tooth.
He wants to wait to see if it heals.
What happens if it doesn't heal?*

Depending upon the severity of the fracture, you may need either a root canal treatment, or your tooth may have to be taken out. Treatment may not be necessary in certain instances where the fracture is minor and gives only slight symptoms.

Your dentist must rely on symptoms to determine the appropriate steps to take. Although x-rays are valuable in diagnosis, sometimes fractures cannot be detected. Other tests, such as tapping on the tooth with a dental instrument and applying cold or heat to the tooth, may help pinpoint the problem.

However, time is the only accurate indicator of the severity of a fracture. Within six to eight weeks your dentist should be able to predict whether your tooth has healed on its own or needs treatment.

Should the pain continue or get stronger, a root canal may be needed to remove the nerve and blood vessels from the inside of your tooth. Even after this procedure, there are no guarantees that the problem will be solved. The tooth may have to be removed later. This may be frustrating for you to hear since you may be losing the tooth. But, any efforts that result in saving a tooth will benefit your health.

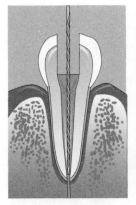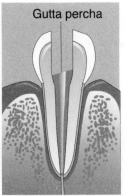

Gutta percha

Chapter 10

Root Canals
Endodontics
- Endo (within)

Pain of infection hurts more than root canal

I'm about to have a root canal done on my front tooth.
What is a root canal? Why is it considered so painful?

A root canal consists of two procedures that eliminate infection affecting nerves and blood vessels in the center of the tooth and its roots.

First the pulp (center area) and tiny canals in the roots are cleaned. An opening in the tooth's surface allows instruments and tiny files to remove debris. Canals in the roots are later filled with a material called "gutta percha."

A root canal refers to both the cleaning and the filling process. Two separate appointments a week apart are usually scheduled to complete the procedure, although in certain instances, it can be finished in one visit.

Continual throbbing or sensitivity to hot and cold foods may be warning signs indicating the need for root canal treatment. A dull toothache and pressure sensitivity when you eat are other signs. Visit your dentist immediately if you have any of these symptoms.

Root canal treatment is often painless, relieving pain caused by bacterial infection. Regular checkups and dental x-rays help detect early infections and guard against root canal problems.

Root Canal Procedure

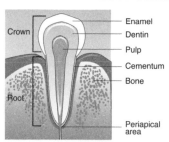

This procedure consists of removing infected nerves and blood from the tooth and its roots.

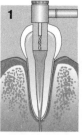

An opening is made in the top of the crown

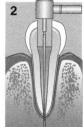

A measurement is taken with an endodontic file.

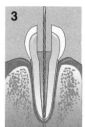

The pulp tissue is removed and root canal is cleaned using rotary instruments.

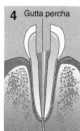

Gutta percha points are coated with a sealing cement.

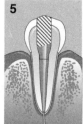

A temporary filling is placed in the opening.

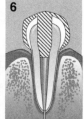

A crown or an amalgam filling is placed on the restoration.

Lack of pain belies the need for root canal

My dentist told me I need a root canal for a tooth that gives me only slight pain. Can something else be done?

Probably not. Your dentist likely based his decision on a careful review of symptoms and tests done on the tooth. An abscess or inflammation at the root of your tooth can be detected with the aid of an x-ray. Signs of infection in the "pulp," or center of the tooth where the nerves and blood supply are located, may also require examination to determine whether the pulp or tooth is alive. If there is little or no response, infection may have damaged this vital part of your tooth beyond recovery.

By postponing the root canal (which involves opening, cleaning and filling the canal in the center of the tooth), a patient risks further decay of the tooth and surrounding teeth and bone. Infection may spread with no warning or discomfort. Symptoms to look for include increased or prolonged sensitivity to heat and cold or to pressure when you bite. If this sensitivity lasts for several minutes, a damaged or re-infected root canal may be the cause.

Other conditions may mimic these symptoms. Trauma to the nerve of the tooth caused by a routine filling may cause a temporary pain called "hyperemia." Other brief periods of tooth sensitivity may indicate other problems your dentist can help diagnose.

Root Canal Test

The root canal operation is done upon the advice of your dentist. There are several ways a dentist can diagnose a root infection or fracture:

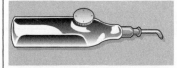

An X-ray is helpful in detecting problems in the root of the tooth, but the electric pulp tester is another safe and effective way to find those trouble spots.

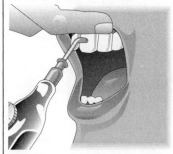

The battery powered EPT sends electric stimulation through the dry tooth. If the nerve is exposed to infection it will respond differently.

Root canal may offer the best decay treatment

My aging mother has gum problems. Now her dentist informs her that one tooth affected by the gum disease needs a root canal. How can gum infection cause a root canal? Can more teeth be infected if the gum problems continue?

When infection reaches the nerve and blood supply of a tooth, root canal treatment is often the only effective way to prevent further damage and eliminate

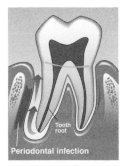

Periodontal infection

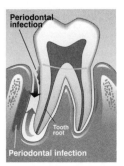

Periodontal infection

Tooth root

Periodontal infection

the infection. In the majority of cases, extensive tooth decay is the cause of this infection. However, periodontal disease can also infect a tooth.

Periodontal Infection

Root canal operations are many times the result of periodontal infections that start in the gums and spread to the tooth root.

As periodontal, or gum-and-bone disease, progresses, infection spreads along the roots of teeth. Eventually it can reach the base or tip of a root where blood vessels and nerves from the body enter a tooth. It is often impossible to see except on x-rays, and usually there is no pain until it reaches the nerves of teeth.

The spread of infection must be stopped or surrounding bone and teeth may deteriorate. Persistent infection may require tooth extraction.

Your dentist will plan a course of treatment that combines root canal and gum-and-bone therapies.

Tooth injuries can have deep-rooted problems

Our son injured one of his front teeth in a bicycling accident. Our dentist told him it was resorbing and may need to be removed. Can the tooth be saved?

Damage by Resorption

Injury to teeth can result in internal or external resorption. This may cause the tooth to be extracted:

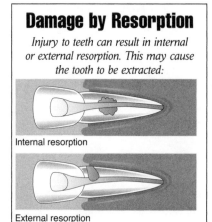

Internal resorption

External resorption

Tooth or root resorption is a slow eating away of the underlying root of a tooth. It may start from the inside by eating away the pulp, or it can begin on the outside and progress inward. Often there is no pain, so resorption can go undetected for a long time.

Internal resorption can result from injury or can occur without an identifiable reason. External resorption may be the result of strong biting forces, tumors or cysts, tooth bleaching, gum disease or trauma.

Effective treatment requires early

diagnosis and prompt attention. Regular x-rays and updated dental-health forms help your dentist detect any resorbing roots and the possible cause. Internal resorption may require replacing a filling, root canal treatment or gum surgery. The tooth may need to be extracted if other treatments are not effective. External resorption that starts at the gumline can be confined by sealing the area with a filling. Resorption beginning below the gums must be treated with special medications and a root canal.

In some cases, the cause cannot be determined. Even with the best of care, some teeth may be lost to resorption.

Tooth may discolor after root canal work

About a year ago, I had a root canal on my front tooth. Now the tooth seems to be getting darker in color. How can the color be corrected?

Root canal treatment involves removal of blood and nerve supplies which are passages for nutrients reaching the tooth. Without these nutrients the tooth becomes brittle and may change in color, frequently getting darker.

After root canal treatment, back teeth usually require onlays or crowns which mask the color changes and protect the tooth from fracturing. Front teeth that are badly broken down or have existing fillings often require similar treatment.

However, front teeth may sometimes be restored with a small filling. Should the tooth later become weakened or change color, it may then require a crown or cap to match the surrounding teeth and to protect it from breaking.

In some cases where just color is a concern, the tooth can be bleached internally. Solutions of bleaching material can be left inside the tooth which will gradually lighten the color over several weeks or months. Once the color matches, the solution can be removed and a permanent filling placed to seal the tooth.

Bleaching may provide a lasting color

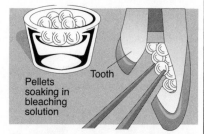

Tooth Discoloration

After a root canal operation, the dead tooth may discolor after a period of time. The tooth can be lightened by internal bleaching. This is how it is done:

Pellets soaking in bleaching solution

Tooth

Cotton pellets soaked in a bleaching solution are inserted into the inside of the tooth.

match. However, some teeth will continue to darken even after the procedure is completed. It is difficult to predict the outcome of such treatments. Your dentist will discuss risks and benefits of your case.

Root canal does not always end tooth woe

I had a root canal done ten years ago and now that molar is starting to hurt. My dentist told me I need something called an "apicoectomy." Can you tell me what that is and why I need it?

Failure of root canal treated teeth occur in the healthiest of patients and with the best of dentists.

Often a process called "percolation" occurs at the root tip of your tooth. Bacteria penetrate the seal at the root tip. If infection seeps back into the root, it may cause discomfort. Removing the root tip or area where this infection has recurred is an "apicoectomy" and is the preferred way to resolve the problem without removing the whole tooth.

This bothersome root tip can be removed by various means. A common method is to make a small hole in your jaw-bone to get access to the root tip. After it is removed, a filling is placed to seal the open end.

An apicoectomy not only removes the source of pain and infection, but allows you to retain the healthy portion of your tooth.

The Apicoectomy

This procedure allows the patient to delete the infected area of a failed root canal operation, while keeping the healthy part of the tooth.

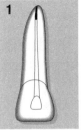
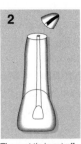
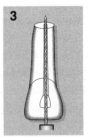
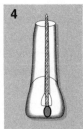

The obstructed or infected root tip.

The root tip is cut off along with the infected or obstructed area.

The canal is then reamed with files.

Trial of master point.

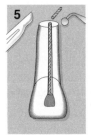
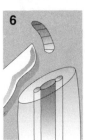
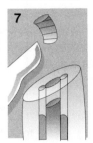
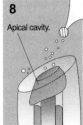
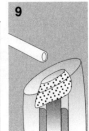

Apical cavity.

Cementation, resection and cold burnishing of master point.

Master point is cut flush with the root end.

Master point pulled from the canal and 3 mm are cut from it and the canal is cemented.

Cement is drilled out and apical cavity prepared.

The seal is placed.

Pain doesn't indicate a failed root canal

My tooth still hurts after a root canal.
Does that mean the nerve wasn't removed completely?
How long should I wait before calling the dentist again?

A root canal is often a painless and simple procedure. However, in some cases, there is discomfort.

Although the nerve is removed, the tooth and surrounding structures may become irritated during the procedure. Slight pain can continue for several days and even weeks until the tooth heals completely.

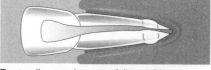

Root callus can be one of the problems confronted after root canal operation.

Root Canal Damage

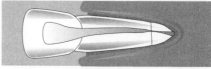

A crack forms from callus.

Pain from root canal operation can be cause for concern if it persists for an extended amount of time:

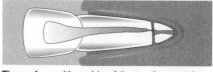

Tissue from either side of the tooth grows into the crack to heal itself.

Sensitivity to biting and chewing is the most common complaint. In such cases, the discomfort usually will subside with time. If the tooth is sensitive to hot or cold liquids or

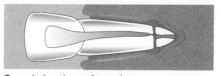

Granulation tissue formation.

throbs spontaneously after a week's time, you should alert your dentist. He or she may advise additional treatment. If the pain does not subside after two weeks, contact your dentist immediately.

Even the best performed root canal treatment runs a risk of failure. Sometimes infection recurs, making efforts to block its path difficult. Fractures in the roots also can complicate treatment.

Keep your dentist aware of any unusual sensation as this may alert him to the need to alter or perform additional work that may prevent ongoing complications.

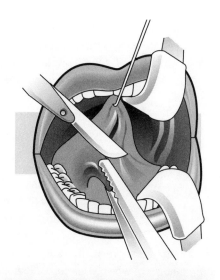

Chapter 11

Oral Surgery

Dentists are not numb to injection techniques

My dentist tried four times to numb my mouth during
my last visit, and still I could feel him working.
I don't want to insult him, but
why can't he do it on the first try?

This situation happens to the best of dentists. Sometimes no matter how good the technique or how cooperative the patient, an anatomic variation in bone structure or nerve location can give this result.

There are, however, racial and individual differences in anatomy that are more prevalent in some populations. These add additional variables to what may be a routine injection. The lower jaw of many Asian races, for example, flares outward more in the area of the ears. This area of bone houses an important nerve which your dentist is aiming for when numbing your lower jaw. A different entry angle and a deeper insertion of the needle help to reach it.

Another difference is the more pronounced degree of jaw and tooth protrusion in Asians, making needle insertion paths change from the Caucasian models often used in dental education. These are only some of the examples that make the science of giving an injection an art.

If you continue to have sensitivity after injections on future appointments, make sure to communicate your anxiety to your dentist. He may want to refer you to a specialist or try a different technique.

Blood pressure check is a safety precaution

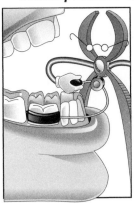

Our dentist wanted to take my father's blood
pressure before having his tooth extracted.
Is this necessary? Why would this be important?

A dentist may elect to take your blood pressure if he suspects that a medical condition can become a problem during a dental procedure. Monitoring blood pressure can thus prevent medical emergencies. Because hypertension often goes unnoticed and undetected, your dentist also may help discover a potential problem.

Oral surgeons and other specialists routinely may

check your blood pressure before scheduling and performing certain surgical procedures. Your family dentist also may take your blood pressure when a problem is noted on your medical or dental health history. Because dental visits can raise blood pressure, your dentist may choose to check it as a safety precaution.

If a problem is detected, your dentist may choose not to perform a procedure. Ongoing problems with elevated blood pressure may require further tests and treatment by a physician. Safety is a top priority for all health procedures and your dentist's request to take your blood pressure is one way to ensure that.

Wisdom teeth removal is wise for your health

I am 30 years old and still have two wisdom teeth.
They don't bother me, but my dentist wants to take them out.
What harm is there to just leave them alone?

Several problems justify the need for removing wisdom teeth. Pockets of gum tissue that can trap food and bacteria, and abnormal development or position of the wisdom teeth are two such conditions that pose risks.

If there are areas around the tooth that collect debris, infection can start and spread with little or no associated pain. Such infection can affect the wisdom tooth or may involve the tooth in front of it. Infection may occur even if the wisdom tooth is not visible above the gumline. Bacteria that collect in back of your last molar tooth can cause a cyst-like growth around the area.

Impaction is a term that refers to the abnormal growth

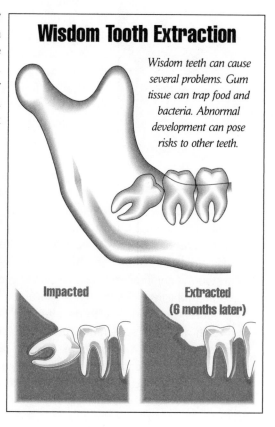

Wisdom Tooth Extraction

Wisdom teeth can cause several problems. Gum tissue can trap food and bacteria. Abnormal development can pose risks to other teeth.

Impacted

Extracted
(6 months later)

and development of a wisdom tooth. Wisdom teeth can develop at odd angles because of their position in the back of the jaw. Sometimes they can butt up against the tooth in front of it.

Teeth normally erupt into the jaw by a forceful pressure that causes a "resorption" or eating away of the bone in front of its path. If there is a tooth in the path, the wisdom tooth may also eat away at it.

In many cases of impaction or infection, there are no serious pain symptoms. However, should these risks be overlooked, continuing infection and danger of losing an additional molar tooth in front of the wisdom tooth may result.

Pulling a tooth can be a complicated task

Recently I had one of my teeth extracted. It took a long time to get it out. Why are some teeth easy to pull and others complicated?

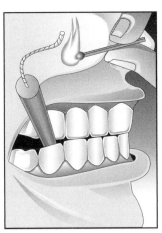

Among the variables that determine the difficulty of extracting teeth are the anatomy of the tooth, the number and shape of the roots, the degree of infection around the tooth, and the attachment of the roots to surrounding bone.

Teeth in front of the mouth generally are easier to remove than molar or back teeth. Molars have two or three roots that are sometimes curved or at differing angles. Such teeth are often first cut in sections so roots can be taken out individually. The anatomy of the teeth and roots varies considerably. Some roots are straight, short and conical while others are twisted, long and flattened.

Infection around a tooth can either make an extraction easier or more difficult, depending on the degree and location of the infection. When infection includes some breakdown of the surrounding bone, extractions may be easier as the tooth is not firmly held by bone. In other cases, however, some infections can pose problems. Sometimes it is difficult to get the tooth numb as bacteria by-products can interfere with the effects of the anesthetic.

Teeth also may sometimes fuse to the surrounding bone. A ligament usually attaches the tooth to bone, but this ligament can degenerate under certain conditions. Teeth fused partially to bone can be quite difficult to remove regardless of other factors. In some cases, surrounding bone has to be removed to take out a root.

Don't extract gauze after tooth is pulled

My son had a tooth extracted a few days ago.
The area is very sore and still bleeds.
Why hasn't it stopped bleeding?

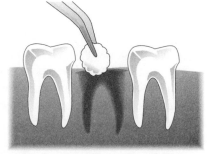

The pain and bleeding are continuing because a blood clot necessary to the healing process has not formed. Often, the longer clot formation takes, the more painful the extraction site remains. Prompt attention and treatment are needed.

Usually after tooth extraction, your dentist places a small pad of gauze over the area and advises you to bite on it for at least an hour. During this time, a clot normally forms and the bleeding stops.

If you rinse, spit, or accidentally move the gauze, bleeding may continue. If so, put another piece of gauze over the extraction site and bite firmly for an hour. If bleeding continues for more than a day or two, obtain medical attention.

Persistent bleeding may be a sign of other health conditions such as hemophilia, liver disease and the overuse of certain medicines. Your dentist is best able to judge whether tests or treatments are needed.

Blood clot is essential to healing of gums

I just had a tooth extracted.
It's been almost two weeks now,
and I still can feel the hole.
It doesn't hurt, but is this normal?

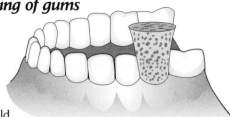

After two weeks, the gums should have healed. If the sensation of the "hole" persists in the next few days, you should visit your dentist.

After removing a tooth, your dentist will usually instruct you to bite hard on a piece of gauze placed over the area. Pressure stops the bleeding and helps to form the clot. This clot is your body's guide to healing; without it, healing will take significantly longer and scar tissue will form.

It is important not to disturb the blood clot while cleaning the area or by spitting or chewing on abrasive foods such as grains and raw vegetables.

Constant irritation may cause a more painful condition called "dry socket," where a clot is unable to form.

Other factors that can delay or aggravate healing include smoking and alcohol consumption. These activities should be avoided for several days after a tooth is removed. Infection caused by bacteria left during extraction of the tooth can aggravate healing and is often painful, requiring treatment with antibiotics.

More serious medical problems affecting the healing process include diseases such as diabetes. Some medical treatments, such as the use of radiation to treat cancer, may reduce blood flow and healing ability.

Traditional sutures are still dentists' choice

Recently I had a tooth extracted before leaving on a trip. I had two stitches which my dentist said would be absorbed so there was no need to come back to have them removed. Is this new stitching better than the old type that the doctor needed to remove?

Suture materials currently used fall into two broad categories: absorbable and non-absorbable. In dentistry these are most commonly represented by gut and silk. Gut sutures or cat gut, as they are often called, are made from the small intestines of sheep or cattle. Thread spun by silkworms to make cocoons is used in silk sutures.

Each type has advantages that benefit a given circumstance and condition. Silk is easy for the dentist to handle and is the most comfortable for the patient. Gut sutures and other absorbable types vary in use and in time of absorption. They are more difficult for your dentist to work with, and usually cause a tissue reaction which can prolong the healing process.

For your situation, your dentist selected an absorbable stitch or suture so you wouldn't need to delay your travel plans with a second visit to remove the stitches.

Normally, the traditional "old type" silk sutures would be removed one week after placement. The gut or absorbable sutures are broken down by body fluids in five to seven days, requiring no follow-up visit for removal.

Silk is still commonly used for closing extraction sites, as are other non-absorbable synthetic fibers.

Surgery frees tongue from pesky attachment

Our 14-week-old son is very fussy while breast-feeding.
Our dentist commented that an attachment from our son's tongue to
the floor of his mouth keeps him from enjoying these feeding times.
Can and should anything be done?

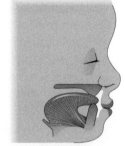

The term *anklyglossia* refers to the attachment of the tongue to the floor of the mouth. Normally, the tongue can freely move in an upward and forward direction. However, this attachment restricts the tongue's movements.

The suckling response for infants with this condition is less gratifying because it prevents them from adequately getting milk from the breast. It is not uncommon for these infants to have slow neonatal weight gain.

Healthy non-restrictive tongue attachments

In many instances, surgical correction can free the tongue from this attachment. The procedure is often simple, and can be completed in a dentist's or pediatrician's office. The impact of such a procedure can influence a child's physiological and psychological development. Even normal speech development may be affected since free movement of the tongue is needed to form certain sounds.

You should discuss this procedure with your dentist or with a specialist should the case be more involved. Because the surgery is often minor, a quick recovery allows a more enjoyable breast-feeding within a few days.

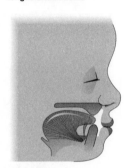

Restrictive tongue attachments

Cleft palate requires vigilant tooth care

One of my nephews has a cleft palate, and we're concerned
about his permanent teeth coming in okay.
What are some of the things we can predict,
and what can be done to keep his teeth straight?

There are a multitude of considerations for an infant or child with cleft palate.

Usually a team of dentists and physicians work together to treat existing problems and to anticipate potential problems. Unmanaged dental conditions can result in severe problems including infection, extensive cavities and tooth misalignment.

Because of the skeletal deformity associated with a palatal cleft, there are problems with the normal eruption of teeth.

Assuming that your nephew has had an operation at an early age to close the palate, there still may be problems with later tooth development and eruption. Incisors and cuspids, or eye teeth, are the teeth most often out of position. The final alignment of these teeth can be corrected by orthodontic and surgical procedures. Surgery to correct the amount of bone needed in that area of clefting is sometimes done in cooperation with the goals of an orthodontist concerned with the final position of the teeth. If certain teeth are missing or beyond repair, implants and prosthetic appliances may aid in restoring the teeth.

A palatal cleft can be a disorder of its own or an indication of a more serious medical condition. Your dentist will want to be assured that any such problems are diagnosed before initiating treatment.

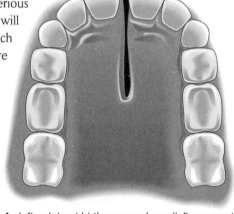

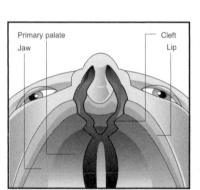

A cleft palate at birth can produce disfigurement in dental adulthood. To correct this birth defect, the palate is surgically rejoined and the teeth are pulled together.

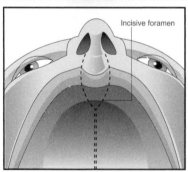

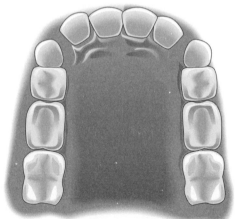

After rejoining the palate, the eye teeth are sometimes separated. This can be corrected with more surgery, implants or orthodontics.

Implants successfully replace missing teeth

My dentist recommended implants to replace the missing teeth in my lower jaw. I'm nervous about the procedure, especially if there may be problems. Should I consider them?

Implants have existed since the 1960s discovery by Professor Pur Ingvar Branemark in Sweden. The present day success rate is between 95-100 percent. New implant materials and improved surgical techniques make this a procedure you should seriously consider.

The Tooth about Implants

Implant fixtures can be a permanent solution to missing teeth. This is how the implant is added:

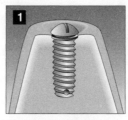

The anchor is drilled into the bone. A cover screw is added and covered with tissue. This allows the tissue to heal and help anchor the fixture.

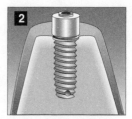

An abutment is added to the fixture after healing period.

Implants are surgically placed metal fixtures, usually made of titanium, that are held in your upper or lower jaw by bone growth that locks onto the implanted device. The implant may be coated with hydroxyapatite, a material matching the mineral content of bone. An implant is commonly

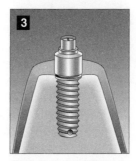

The fixture is then added and screwed in from the top.

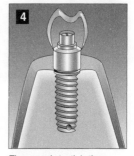

The ceramic tooth is then cemented to the anchor.

shaped like a simple cylindrical screw. The number of missing teeth being replaced as well as the amount of bone loss are some of the factors that determine the number and type of fixtures that will be used.

Your dentist will review many aspects of your dental and medical health to ensure the best result. Implants work in most cases, giving you a feeling of having your own teeth.

Speech problem can be treated surgically

My trouble with speaking is partially caused by my tongue. It doesn't move around normally, and I can't even touch the roof of my mouth. Can anything be done, and if so, would I be able to speak better?

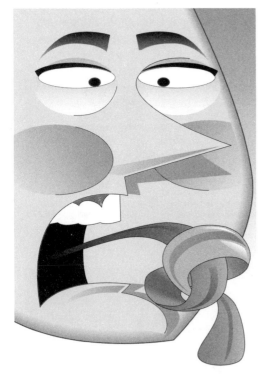

Restrictive muscle attachments to the lips and tongue can cause speech problems. Sometimes there is an attachment from the tip of the tongue to the lower lip or to the floor of the mouth. This prevents free movement of the tongue. Words such as "Thursday" become

Muscular tongue attachments can sometimes be too short to allow free movement, posing a problem for speech

impossible to say without touching the tongue to the roof of the mouth. In some other cases, there are muscle attachments from the lips to the gums that can restrict lip movements. Formation of words such as "morning" are difficult to pronounce when the lips cannot move freely.

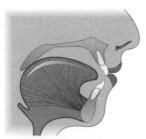

Healthy non-restrictive tongue attachments

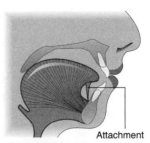

Attachment

Restrictive tongue attachments

Treatment includes cutting the muscle attachment either partially or completely to allow free movement. The procedures are easy and can be done by your family dentist or an oral surgeon.

Tongue attachments can hinder movement, posing a problem for speech. Out-patient care can remedy this problem. Here's how:

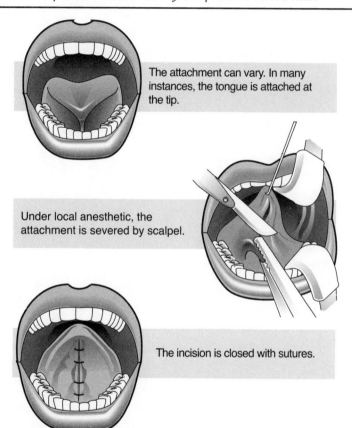

The attachment can vary. In many instances, the tongue is attached at the tip.

Under local anesthetic, the attachment is severed by scalpel.

The incision is closed with sutures.

Some muscle attachments can move teeth in addition to restricting the movement of soft tissue. For example, there are instances when a muscle attachment from the lips to the gums at the base of the front teeth can cause the teeth to separate. After the teeth have moved apart, there are unnatural spaces which, besides being unsightly, can cause other speech problems. In such cases, after the muscle attachment is separated, an orthodontist may need to move the teeth back together.

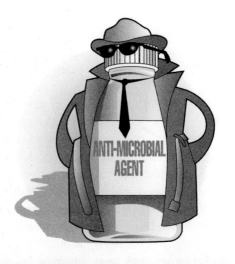

Chapter 12

Medicines for Teeth

Antibiotics used to treat gum disease

*As part of my treatment for gum disease, my dentist
has recommended that I take antibiotics for about one month.
My stomach usually bothers me when I take antibiotics.
Isn't there another way of treating this?*

Many factors influence periodontal disease and the likelihood of any treatment working well. Short-term antibiotics are frequently prescribed to control bacteria. Systemic or local antibiotics are useful as a temporary measure to control infection. Usually oral tablets or capsules are given. Some newer techniques use time-released antibiotics placed directly around the infection site.

If your stomach aches after taking antibiotics for a long duration, let your dentist know. Eating foods such as yogurt and cheese with good bacteria to replace those destroyed by an antibiotic can limit stomach pain. However, do not eat bacteria-rich foods within an hour of taking an antibiotic.

Keep your dentist up to date on medications you take. They may inhibit the effectiveness of antibiotics.

Antibiotics can hinder the pill's effectiveness

*I was recently treated for a dental abscess.
On the health form was a question asking
if I was taking birth-control pills.
Why is this information important?*

After draining an abscess, a dentist often prescribes. antibiotics to clear out the bacteria that caused the infection. Some antibiotics may interfere with the function of birth-control pills, a fact that the ten million women in this country who take birth-control pills should know.

The association came up recently in two cases where unplanned pregnancies were linked to the reduced effect of birth-control pills due to antibiotic use.

The pill can fail for other reasons. In some instances, women fail to follow the regimen, and in a small fraction of the cases, the pill doesn't work at all. But because of the documented association, if you are taking birth-control pills, be sure your dentist knows.

Agents help combat tooth decay bacteria

We seem to have a lot of tooth decay in our family.
Our parents tell us and our children that we have
soft teeth. Recently, our dentist gave us a gel
to use with something called chlorhexidine.
Is this effective and how does it work?

The treatment of tooth decay has changed
dramatically over the past ten years. Your family
dentist traditionally concentrated on removing
decay with a dental drill, then restoring the area with
a filling. Primary emphasis was placed on brushing, flossing, and dietary changes,
all of which help prevent continued tooth decay. Now tooth decay is viewed
more as an infectious and transmissible disease. In addition to the traditional
methods to control it, anti-microbial agents may be needed and prescribed by
your dentist. These gels are combined with other preventive measures such as
fluoride coatings, rinses and sealants.

Chlorhexidine is one of the more common anti-microbial agents used to
control plaque, tooth decay and gum disease. Your dentist may prescribe it as a
rinse or gel depending on the degree and type of oral infection.

Bacteria in the mouth have been shown to be transmitted either by direct
contact such as kissing or by indirect contact through shared cups, utensils or
toothbrushes. The terms soft and hard teeth have no meaning in current-day
dentistry. Rather, finding the source of tooth decay and treating its cause is the
goal of modern dental care. Preventive measures using sealants, fluoride and
anti-microbial agents all may help to stop the spread of bacteria which cause
tooth decay.

Acupuncture can be applied in dentistry

Can acupuncture work for dental treatment?
My friend is convinced that acupuncture
helped her with the jaw pain she was having.
How does it work and what types of
procedures can it be used for?

Acupuncture is one of the oldest medical therapies.
Traced from its roots in China, acupuncture is based on

establishing and maintaining the flow of life energy or *chi*. This energy circulates through the bodies of living organisms in patterns of meridians or lines of force. Points along these meridians are selected for the insertion of fine needles, which release any blockage along this line of flow. Healing occurs when obstructed flow is restored. Western medicine believes that body-healing compounds such as endorphins, are released with the application of acupuncture needles.

Because meridians link many organs within the body, problems in one area may signal difficulty in a related organ along the same meridian. The kidney meridian, for example, is linked with bone development in the jaw, and the spleen and stomach meridian are linked with the gums.

Applications in dentistry range from toothaches to stress-management and healing. Depending on the type and source of pain, a dentist can work in conjunction with an acupuncturist to treat a patient.

Drug combinations can cause new side effects

I was surprised during my recent dental visit when my dentist said that I shouldn't take the antibiotic erythromycin for an infection because I was taking Seldane for my allergies. Can you explain why the concern since I've never had a problem with erythromycin before?

Many drugs, when taken together produce affects that neither alone can cause. Such interactions have become so complex that new side effects are as common as new drugs on the market. Seldane is an antihistamine commonly used to relieve hay fever. Recent studies indicate that people taking Seldane and erythromycin can have severe cardiac arrhythmias. Because of the possible serious interaction between these two commonly prescribed drugs, dentists and physicians have avoided their concurrent use.

Your doctor will have current reports available so that such potential problems can be avoided. Be sure to fill out your complete health history form when visiting your dentist.

With current, updated information your dentist can better advise you about drugs that you can use to safely treat your dental needs.

Medicine's side effects felt on empty stomach

*My dentist recently gave me some pain killers
after treating my abscessed tooth.
I've been feeling nauseous and tired.
Would it be better to just stop taking them?*

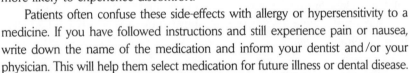

Pain killers, or "analgesics," are sometimes the only way to reduce toothache pain. Many have side effects. Among the more common problems are stomach discomfort and nausea.

To help prevent these side-effects, always take pain medication after eating. If you haven't eaten for several hours, you are more likely to experience discomfort.

Patients often confuse these side-effects with allergy or hypersensitivity to a medicine. If you have followed instructions and still experience pain or nausea, write down the name of the medication and inform your dentist and/or your physician. This will help them select medication for future illness or dental disease.

Another thing to consider: it is a mistake to wait until pain comes on before taking pain medication. The body requires considerably more medicine to counteract existing pain. In fact, some researchers believe it is better to take pain medication before or during certain dental visits. If the medication is already in your system, you are less likely to experience subsequent pain.

Do not drink alcohol while taking prescription pain medicines and avoid any additional medications without your doctor's approval. Also, do not drive or use machinery. Such medicines can distort perception and cloud judgment.

Stopping the bacteria that cause bone loss

*My husband recently went to a periodontist to have his gum
disease treated. In addition to the surgery, he has been placed
on antibiotics for a long time. Why does he need to take
the antibiotics for weeks after the surgery?
Are there alternatives to this prolonged antibiotic use?*

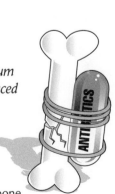

Certain medicines and drugs have continued to show benefits for people suffering from periodontal or gum-and-bone disease. There are two broad categories of these medications. The first includes antibiotics to prevent the spread of bacteria that cause gum-and-bone degeneration. The second type includes NSAIDS, or non-steroidal anti-inflammatory drugs, which are effective in preventing bone loss. These drugs used in combination with traditional surgery, have proved to be beneficial, especially in cases where the surgery is recurring.

Antibiotics like tetracycline can be given orally or placed directly in the diseased-tissue area. More techniques are being developed to place the medicine directly on the tissue since there are drawbacks to long-term use of antibiotics in the body.

Tetracycline taken orally kills many of the body's good bacteria as well as the specific microbe affecting the diseased tissue. In addition, when taken in the body, very little of its effect gets to the specific diseased area. For these reasons, direct application of antibiotics to the gum tissue is used more frequently.

NSAIDS, like a compound called flurbiprofen, have been shown to inhibit the loss of bone in patients with periodontal disease. Although these drugs are in the initial phases of clinical use, they may be a helpful addition to conventional surgery.

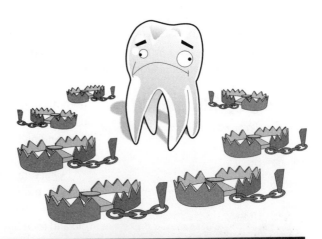

Chapter 13

Medical Conditions with Dental Consequences

Tongue may be a site of cancer detection

My dentist has me stick out my tongue during routine checkups.
Is he checking my throat or my tongue?

Your dentist is checking your tongue. The side of the tongue is one of the more common sites for a form of oral cancer called squamous cell carcinoma. This type of cancer accounts for 91 percent of all oral malignancies.

Hung by the Tongue

In 91% of oral cancer cases, the tongue is involved

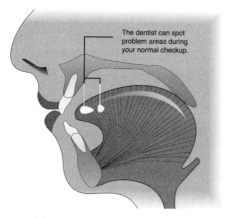

The dentist can spot problem areas during your normal checkup.

Chances are good he will find nothing unusual. But for 30,000 of us this year, oral cancer will be a new finding in our dental or medical record.

Oral cancer occurs predominantly in older men. Ninety-five percent of the cases are in people over 40 years old and men have twice the chance of being diagnosed with the disease. The male to female ratio in the 1950s was considerably higher at six-to-one, but most researchers feel the gap has narrowed due to the increase of women smokers.

If suspicious growths are found, a biopsy may be scheduled to determine the presence of cancer. Oral cancers typically appear as white patches that usually go unnoticed by the patient. In most cases, a small piece of the affected area is removed for analysis. Most of these cancers can be detected at an early stage and treated with a high degree of success.

White patch alerts smokers to cancer

I'm a cigar smoker. My dentist told me about an area
in my mouth that has a white patch. He said it's okay now,
but may develop into cancer. Do these ever go away?

If you stop smoking, the patch may go away if it has not already developed into cancer. If you continue to smoke, you live with the daily risk of that white patch becoming cancerous.

Leukoplakia is the name given to such an area not identified as any other disease. The patches are usually found on the underside of the tongue or floor of the mouth and can vary in size and appearance. Constant irritation of the area from smoking leads to this change and in three to five percent of the cases to cancer.

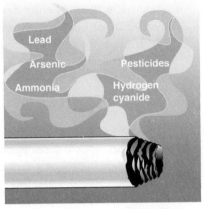

Tobacco smoke contains some very toxic agents including lead, arsenic, hydrogen cyanide, ammonia and pesticides, just to name a few. Continual exposure to these gases and chemicals over a long period may cause cancer. In addition, if you have sores or ulcers, they are less likely to heal when being exposed to cigar or cigarette smoke. Often, after a tooth extraction, your dentist strongly recommends that you not smoke because healing will be delayed. Gum disease can also be aggravated by continued exposure to cigar and cigarette smoke and smokeless tobacco.

Heart patients should delay dental work

My dad has heart problems. About two months ago, he had a myocardial infarction. There is a tooth that has been bothering him, but he doesn't want to see the dentist for a while. How soon after the myocardial infarction can he visit a dentist? Is there any danger in delaying the visit?

Dental treatment should be delayed for three to six weeks for patients recovering from myocardial infarction. During this period, the heart muscle often is electrically unstable. Stress from some dental procedures may cause additional heart problems. Your body's epinephrine can increase as much as twenty-fold when under stress from dental procedures. Even after several months of recovery time, anesthetics containing epinephrine should be avoided. Only when your cardiologist has evaluated the condition as being stable should such anesthetics be used.

Other heart conditions warrant concern. For example, patients undergoing heart bypass surgery or those having certain arrhythmias or irregular heart beats should be evaluated before dental treatment. In general, for three months following major heart surgery, routine visits to the dentist should be delayed. Your dentist will consult with your cardiologist as each person and surgery has individual concerns.

In certain instances, a toothache can take precedence over the risks of post-surgical heart problems. Treatment of abscesses and severe infections associated with teeth and surrounding bone should not be delayed.

Patients with heart problems should provide a detailed medical history to their dentists. Special considerations of antibiotic use and anesthetic selection may be critical in providing dental care.

Anesthetics may cause heart to race

During my last dental visit, I felt my heart racing for about a minute after an anesthetic injection. The experience scared me.
What causes this and how can it be avoided?

Local anesthetics used in dentistry commonly contain an agent called a vasoconstrictor. These agents have three functions. The first is to increase the duration of the anesthetic. The second is to slow your body's absorption rate because too much anesthesia can be toxic. And last, anesthetics reduce the amount of bleeding in an area.

The feeling of a racing heart may be associated with a vasoconstrictor agent in the local anesthetic. People with cardiovascular disease may be particularly sensitive. Anesthetics with a high concentration of a vasoconstrictor are more likely to result in such a reaction. For this reason, your dentist tries to use an anesthetic with a minimal amount of the agent.

Sometimes during routine injections, anesthetics can directly enter a blood vessel. This may also stimulate the sensation of a racing heart or fast pulse. Because blood vessels often run next to nerves, it's possible for your dentist to accidentally inject anesthetic into a blood vessel. He avoids such risk by aspirating, or pulling back on the syringe, to check if blood is present.

Oral bacteria can also endanger the heart

I have an artificial heart valve which was placed several years ago.
Since then, my dentist has prescribed antibiotics before dental cleanings.
Last week, however, he completed a small filling
and said the antibiotic was unnecessary.
How does a dentist determine when you need the medication?

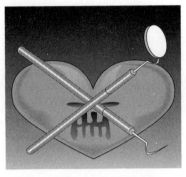

Pre-medication for dental treatment is commonly given to people suffering from heart conditions. Without antibiotics, oral bacteria released during dental cleanings and gum surgery could cause *subacute bacterial endocarditis*, a serious infection of the heart requiring hospitalization and often surgery. The illness starts when bacteria, dislodged from teeth and gums, flows through the bloodstream to other parts of the body.

For most people, the amount of bacteria can be easily handled by the body's defense systems. But for patients with certain heart conditions, bacterial plaques or collections can form in the blood vessels of the heart.

Dentists often consult with physicians to evaluate medication needs. If your dentist works on a small filling on an edge of the tooth away from the gumline, the risk is generally minimal.

Stomach acid can damage your teeth

Ever since my stomach ulcers were diagnosed several months ago,
I've noticed some of my teeth are
sensitive. I brush and floss regularly,
especially if there is an acid taste in
my mouth. What else can I do?

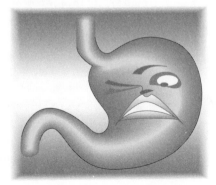

Stomach acid from ulcers can affect your teeth. If you are aware of acid contents or vapors in your mouth, damage to the teeth is likely occurring. Acid gradually erodes tooth structures.

Because the acid comes from the stomach, the back surfaces of your teeth are affected more than the front surfaces.

Brushing the teeth after exposure to stomach acid is damaging. Abrasion from the brushing with concentrated acid accelerates the wear of the tooth surface. Sensitivity of the teeth is caused from this erosion of acid and abrasion from brushing.

To prevent continuing tooth wear, the acid should be neutralized with a basic compound. A mixture of baking soda and water is good to rinse with before brushing. Only after the acid is neutralized is it advisable to brush your teeth. Keeping regular checkups with your dentist will help monitor your condition.

Alcohol can ravage drinkers' teeth and gums

My husband is a recovering alcoholic. Could his drinking have done any damage to his teeth and gums?

Alcohol affects many parts of the mouth and is associated with many diseases. Oral cancer is the most serious dental problem for people who drink heavily. Alcohol does not directly cause cancer, but cancer-causing agents are more likely to induce malignancies in people who are heavy drinkers.

Chronic alcohol use also can affect the health of the gums. Periodontal disease often is more difficult to control in an alcoholic patient. Likewise, open sores and sites of tooth extraction do not heal as fast. Blood clots allow tissue to heal normally. For heavy drinkers, the clot-forming mechanism is impaired. Without rapid blood-clot formation, even minor gum and tooth surgery can be serious.

Teeth are affected by alcohol, which can erode their outer surfaces. This wearing away of teeth is directly linked to another symptom of heavy drinking: vomiting. Acids in the stomach can cause premature wearing of the outer enamel layer of teeth. Erosion of the biting edges and surfaces along the palate of upper teeth is common in such cases. Crowns are often needed to protect against further wear and tooth fractures.

Since your husband is recovering from alcoholism, his oral health is likely to return.

Avoid mouthwash if on a low sodium diet

I've heard that the sodium content in some mouthwashes can be harmful for certain people. Is that true, and, if so, why?

For most of us, foods rich in sodium are a welcome addition to our diet. But there are certain medical conditions where average amounts of sodium can be dangerous. For those people on a low-sodium diet, something new may be added to the list of things to avoid: mouthwash. If you suffer from hypertension, obesity and renal disease, among others, you may want to watch the ingredient label on mouth rinses.

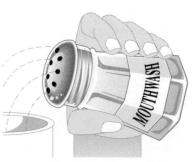

If you are watching the sodium in your diet, you should also be carefully reading labels on all containers. If you have a normal diet, the sodium in mouthwashes has no measurable effect on your body. But for those with certain medical problems, continued use is cause for concern. Researchers warn that if you are on a low-sodium diet, you should avoid the use of mouthwashes and consult with your physician or dentist about a substitute.

Sinus infections can be the root of toothaches

My dentist says my aching tooth is probably caused by a sinus infection. Is this common? How can a dentist tell it is a sinus problem, not a tooth problem?

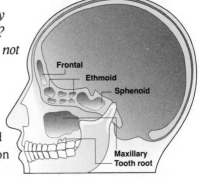

Infections of teeth and sinuses are sometimes interconnected. An aching tooth can be caused by an infection in and around that tooth, or from a sinus infection near the tooth, or from both sources.

Sinuses are large air cavities located in your upper jaw above your upper teeth. Membranes that line these cavities can become infected. If the roots of upper teeth near these sinuses are close to such an infection, you may experience a toothache.

To locate the source of pain, a dentist will usually take an x-ray to look for infected roots. If the roots appear normal, he or she will look at how close the sinus cavity is to the base of the roots and seek evidence of an infected sinus.

The tooth also may be tested for sensitivity by tapping lightly on the surface and exposing it to hot and cold temperatures. If a tooth is very sensitive, it's likely the tooth is the source of the problem. A continual dull ache or throbbing sensation, combined with a lack of response to these tests, may point to a sinus infection.

Treatment for a sinus infection includes antibiotics and decongestants. In some cases, your dentist may refer you to an ear-nose-and-throat specialist.

Eating disorders can show signs on teeth

Can a dentist tell if someone has anorexia? We are puzzled by suspicions that our dentist has concerning our daughter. Apparently her teeth are worn in such a way that this may be a likely cause.

Eating disorders such as anorexia and bulimia can often be detected by your dentist. Signs and patterns of excessive wear on the teeth may indicate such disorders. Typically, the inside surfaces of the teeth have wear from stomach acids that are continually exposed to these areas. Often these individuals drink excessive amounts of sugar-free carbonated drinks, adding to the degree of tooth wear. Depending on the amount of time that these beverages are in contact with the teeth, wear on the outside surfaces may be evident.

Treatment must involve all aspects of the disorder to be effective. Fluoride rinses, extensive restorative work, including fillings, crowns and porcelain veneers, may all be needed to restore dental health. Excessive consumption of carbonated beverages needs to be controlled. Psychological support of family and all treating health care providers needs to be constant. Even the best dental care eventually will fail without such support.

Diabetics are prone to gum and bone infections

My mother is diabetic and has a continual problem with gum disease. Is this common, and what can be done to treat or prevent further infection in her mouth?

There is a strong association that links diabetes with gum disease. Recent findings by the National Institutes of Health show that diabetics are more likely to have ongoing gum and bone infections with serious complications.

Diabetes affects 12 million Americans with an added 600,000 new cases each year. The disease is a metabolic disorder which is broadly classified in two categories: juvenile onset and adult onset. The first requires insulin therapy, which helps nutrients enter a person's cells. Adult onset diabetes is more variable in its symptoms and does not always require insulin therapy. Both forms and the variations in between them are associated with periodontal or gum disease. Juvenile onset diabetes is a more severe form of the disease and thus in later years is often associated with more destructive gum and bone infections.

These ongoing infections destroy the structure of a tooth's foundation. Without bone support and gum health, teeth become loose and are prone to infection. Diabetics like your mother should take several precautions to limit ongoing gum disease. Regular and even frequent tooth cleanings can help monitor the progression of the infection.

Taking the recommended insulin doses and following dietary recommendations prescribed by your physician will help control the disease and, thus, the mouth infections that are linked to it. Those with advanced gum infections and no established cause should also follow through carefully with a medical and dental work-up. Sometimes adult onset diabetes is diagnosed after treating ongoing episodes of periodontal infection.

Researchers believe that diabetes predisposes an individual to a lower resistance in his or her gum and bone tissues, allowing infection to occur and spread more easily. Only by aggressively treating the disease and monitoring the diabetes can these infections be controlled.

Jaw arthritis sufferers find options for relief

A dental specialist told me that I have osteoarthritis in my jaw joint. Can you explain more about what causes this and the best way to relieve the pain? It still bothers me.

Signs of arthritis can be found in 97 percent of Americans between the ages of 40 and 60. It's marked by a deterioration of body tissues, particularly bone and cartilage. Swelling, pain, redness and heat are frequent symptoms. Osteoarthritis is one of the most common forms of arthritis and is often found in jaw x-rays. Many people with osteoarthritis in the jaw joint function normally, while others experience muscle tenderness and pain when moving the joint.

There are two different forms of osteoarthritis. Primary osteoarthritis is a gradual "wear and tear" of a joint that builds up over a long time. Secondary arthritis occurs by direct injury to the joint, such as infection or bone trauma.

Osteoarthritis in the Jaw

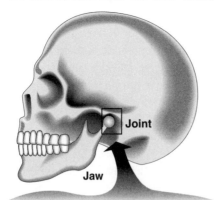

"Bruxism" (tooth grinding) and clenching (biting down firmly) are two of the most frequent causes of osteoarthritis. Stresses from tooth grinding dry out the lubricating fluids within the joint. When component parts of a joint then move against each other, abnormal friction causes gradual erosion of the normal bone and cartilage contours. Muscles around the joint also tense up in response to this damage.

There are several factors you can control to limit the stress on an inflamed jaw joint. If you experience pain when eating, confine your diet to softer foods. Moist heat packs and massage also help relieve muscle stiffness around the joint.

Your dentist can choose more appropriate treatments after examining your jaw and joint. If a faulty bite is the source

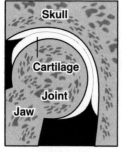

A healthy joint consists of bone and cartilage that allows smooth motion.

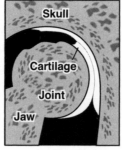

Cartilage is eaten away by arthritis and bone is allowed to wear down causing inflammation.

of your joint pain, an orthotic or a plastic splint can be custom-molded to fit between your teeth. These distribute biting forces evenly throughout the mouth. Orthotics are made for people who clench or grind their teeth since they relieve pressure within the joint.

Medications such as steroids, anti-inflammatory drugs and pain medications may provide additional help to relieve muscle and joint pain. In severe cases where pain persists, surgery may be required to alter the bone or cartilage contour and remove degenerating tissue.

Osteoporosis affects all bones, including the jaw

Can osteoporosis affect your jaw-bone? My dentures seem to loosen faster than those of other people I know. What can I do to prevent or correct this bone loss?

By the age of 60, one third of all white women in the United States are afflicted by osteoporosis. This degenerative bone condition affects all bones, including your jaw-bone, accelerating bone loss or resorption.

Teeth can become loose as the bone supporting them diminishes. Likewise, the bony ridge on which dentures rest also resorbs, causing these appliances to prematurely loosen.

Dentists play an important role in helping to diagnose and predict oral problems of osteoporosis. Often, more frequent visits are helpful to predict and treat problems caused from loosened teeth and resorbed bone. To correct loose dentures, your dentist may reline the denture with an acrylic or soft material that will compensate for the amount of bone loss underneath the denture. More frequent relines may be necessary as bone loss is more progressive for those with osteoporosis.

Normally, lining materials can last for several years. For those denture wearers with osteoporosis, a reline may be necessary as often as every year. The eventual loss of bone mass in such individuals can exceed 75 percent and progresses at different rates for each individual. As much as 50 percent of bone mass can be lost before osteoporosis is even diagnosed.

Dryness may indicate Sjogren's Syndrome

My wife was told recently that she may have Sjogren's Syndrome. What is it and what can be done to treat it?

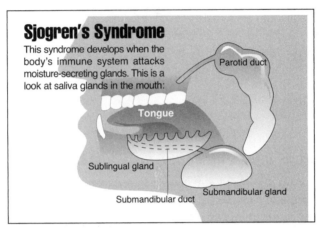

Sjogren's Syndrome

This syndrome develops when the body's immune system attacks moisture-secreting glands. This is a look at saliva glands in the mouth:

Parotid duct

Tongue

Sublingual gland

Submandibular duct

Submandibular gland

Sjogren's (pronounced "show-grins") Syndrome, or auto-immune exocrinopathy, develops when the body's immune system attacks moisture-secreting glands.

Symptoms include dry mouth and eyes and a generalized dryness in many other areas of the body. Of the 660,000 people in the United States who know they have Sjogren's Syndrome, 90 percent are women, and most are post-menopausal.

Many others are unaware of their condition, partly because patients do not report all their symptoms. For example, when a patient tells a dentist about a dry mouth, but not about dry eyes, the dentist is likely to consider causes that are more common than Sjogren's.

Sjogren's Syndrome affects the mouth in many ways. Patients are more prone to tooth decay and gum infection since the affected glands that normally produce a protective barrier of saliva are impaired.

Difficulty chewing or limited jaw movement may be experienced, which may reflect joint pain throughout the body. Half of all Sjogren's patients also have arthritis.

Treatment includes frequent visits to both a dentist and an ophthalmologist. Other specialists may be needed to provide complete treatment for other areas of the body. Because the underlying cause is not well understood, treating the symptoms is the best method to control it.

To learn more, contact the Sjogren's Syndrome Foundation, 382 Main St., Port Washington, NY 11050.

Fixing your smile may affect your new knee

I've had a total knee replacement and am concerned about it becoming infected. Is it true that dental procedures can cause infection in artificial joints?

Many prosthetic devices must be guarded from infection – and one source of infection is bacteria spread through the bloodstream during dental surgery. There has long been an association between dental infection and prosthetic heart valves, which are more likely to trap bacteria, resulting in serious heart infection. To minimize the risk, an antibiotic may be given during dental procedures.

The association between dental work and infection in prosthetic joints is less clear. Some orthopedic surgeons favor using antibiotics prior to certain dental procedures but the American Academy of Oral Medicine has determined there is insufficient scientific evidence to support making such a practice routine. Current guidelines from a joint commission of the American Dental Association and the American Academy of Orthopedic Surgeons state that unless there are certain medical conditions present there is no need for pre-medication two years after prosthetic joint surgery.

Cases may vary, and so you should ask your physician and/or dentist for a recommendation which will depend on your prosthesis and medical condition, and the dental treatment.

Complex saliva vital to general well-being

I have dry mouth from a drug that helps my hypertension. Since taking it, I've developed sores at the corners of my mouth and have problems eating. My dentist informed me that I may develop new cavities as well. Are there any other problems that can occur that I should be warned about?

There are approximately 430 drugs prescribed today, for a variety of illnesses, that have a side effect of decreasing saliva production.

Although saliva may appear to be a simple lubricating fluid for the mouth, it is quite complex. There are hundreds of components each with functions that have been researched.

Saliva fights certain microbes and maintains the balance of bacteria in the mouth. Without saliva, the mouth is more prone to bacterial infection. Besides the symptoms you describe, there are many others that may develop as a direct result of dry mouth. For example, you may have difficulty chewing and tasting food. A burning or tingling sensation in the tongue has also been described by some people. Speaking can be more difficult. Dry mouth, often accompanied by dry nose and throat, also makes breathing more strained.

Saliva also contains minerals that replenish those lost from teeth. Without such a source of minerals, you are more prone to tooth decay as your dentist described.

Digestive enzymes contained in saliva begin breaking down food in the mouth, preparing them for further digestion in the stomach. Without these enzymes the stomach may be overloaded with digestive work and can develop ulcers. Saliva also contains materials to keep mucous membranes like your gums and cheeks healthy and lubricated.

Because of these various functions, many of the daily chores of life can become painful. Your awareness can help alert your physician or dentist of ways to treat these symptoms. Simple precautions, like keeping a glass of water by your bedside to help with a dried throat or mouth, can help. If the problems that develop from such a drug outweigh the benefits of the medication, your physician or dentist may suggest an alternative drug.

Alzheimer's patients suffer oral problems

Our grandmother has Alzheimer's Disease and among other concerns,
we worry about her teeth. She is getting more cavities now.
What can we do to help her?

An estimated four million Americans suffer from Alzheimer's Disease, the most common form of dementia in the elderly. Both the incapacitating nature of their disease and the decreased function of their salivary glands cause oral problems such as gum disease and an increased number of cavities in Alzheimer's patients.

If your grandmother has difficulty brushing and flossing, you may want to help her. In addition, mechanical brushes and sprays and rinses containing the compound chlorhexidine are helpful.

Because those with Alzheimer's have decreased salivary flow, they are more prone to tooth decay. Saliva helps wash away plaque, bacteria and buffers acids, which, if not controlled, can make a tooth more susceptible to decay.

Frequent rinsing with water or use of a dental irrigator such as a Water Pik can help wash away food debris. Application of fluoride gels on the outer exposed surfaces by the gumline of the teeth can also help prevent ongoing decay.

There are simple tests that can help you and your grandmother monitor how well you are cleaning the teeth.

Changes in the mouth may warn of AIDS

I've tested positive for HIV (human immunodeficiency virus), and am wondering if this is causing my gums to bleed and appear puffy?

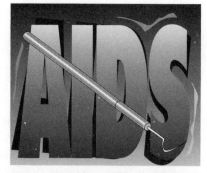

A progressive form of gum and bone disease is often associated with HIV infection or AIDS. The smooth, light pink normal gums become puffy, turn dark red or gray, and recede. If usual cleanings or gum surgery do not reverse these symptoms, the HIV virus is often suspected.

Gum ulcers and rapid unexplained bone loss are also possible. Dentists may recommend testing for the HIV virus to patients who experience these unexplained indicators of periodontal disease.

Because you have indicated that you are HIV positive, routine dental cleanings and good oral hygiene may not be sufficient to stop your gum and bone disease. Medications, surgery and laser treatment are often needed.

Other changes in the mouth associated with HIV infection include Kaposi's sarcoma, a malignant tumor that resembles a blood clot and is usually found on the palate or gums. The fungal condition, candidiasis, or thrush, in an otherwise healthy person can also indicate HIV infection.

Repeat bouts of more common oral infections such as herpes, warts, aphthous ulcers and elongated taste buds may also be warning signs of AIDS. These conditions have other causes, but repeated studies linking them with the HIV virus should prompt a visit to your dentist.

Youths would be wise to snuff out bad habit

Our 14-year-old son uses snuff during his baseball games. We are trying to get him to stop, but he won't. Can you explain the risks?

Approximately 16 million Americans use smokeless tobacco. According to the American Academy of Head and Neck Surgery, three million users are under age 21, and 16 percent of the males between 12 and 17 years old use smokeless tobacco.

There are two types of smokeless tobacco, those sold as pouches, called plugs, and finely ground tobacco known as snuff. Users place a small amount between their cheek and gums.

Although proponents of smokeless tobacco say the product is safe, research conducted by the American Cancer Society and the Advisory Committee to the Surgeon General revealed that continued use of smokeless tobacco can lead to oral cancer. A 1986 Surgeon General report concluded that there is a dramatic increase in the risk of cancer of the gums and cheek among long-term users of smokeless tobacco.

Nitrosamines are the main cancer-causing agents found in smokeless tobacco. One pouch of smokeless tobacco has nearly ten times the nitrosamines as a single cigarette. Several years ago, the Food and Drug Administration banned the sale of bacon containing a small fraction of the nitrosamines found in smokeless tobacco.

If your family dentist notices any changes on your son's gums or cheeks, such as the appearance of a white patch, these are likely precancerous.

The effects of smokeless tobacco are reversible if your son stops his habit before these changes occur. Precancerous signs may or may not be reversed.

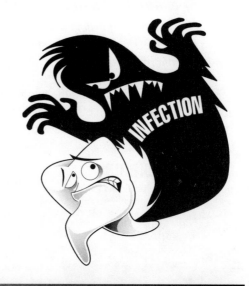

Chapter 14

Oral Infections

Oral self-exam assists in early cancer detection

Is there a method for performing a self-exam for oral cancer? I've been smoking for over 20 years and am concerned about things to check for when I look into my mouth.

Smoking and alcohol use are the two most common factors which lead to oral cancer. The combination of both is lethal, so your concern is justified. Over 30,000 Americans will be diagnosed with oral cancer this year. Approximately 10,000 will die from it.

Self-Exams

These are techniques in self-examination for cancer.

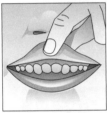

Use thumb and forefinger to examine under upper and lower lips.

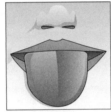

For tongue exams, begin by sticking tongue straight out and checking surface.

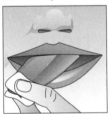

Using a piece of gauze, pull the tongue from side to side, checking for lesions on either side.

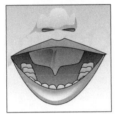

Touching the tongue to the top of the mouth allows you to examine underneath.

A self-exam is easy to perform and may make early detection possible.

The most common area for oral cancer to appear is on the lips. You should look in the mirror at your upper and lower lips, and examine both the outer and inner surfaces for any sores or colored areas. Then check for any lumps or swellings by holding the lip between the thumb and index finger, and moving along the entire lip surface.

The second most common area is the side of the tongue. To examine the tongue, stick it straight out and first examine the top surface. Then, using a piece of gauze, hold the tongue and move it from right to left to examine both sides.

Finally, touch the tongue to the roof of your mouth to see areas underneath. Any discoloration or swelling in any of these areas should be noted.

The floor of the mouth should also be examined. Place one finger directly on the floor of the mouth and one finger outside of the mouth under your chin. Pressing both fingers lightly against each other, you can detect any swellings. Again, move the fingers together so that the entire floor of the mouth is examined.

Check for any color changes or sores in the cheeks and gums. By using the thumb and index finger of one hand, you will be able to detect any growth in the cheeks.

The side of the face and neck area should be looked at and touched. Look for any sores or warts and moles that may have changed in color or size.

Inform your dentist of any changes. If an old sore looks unusual, or a new sore develops, you should make an appointment with your dentist. Remember, often the most serious forms of oral cancer are not painful.

Check immediately for any growths in the mouth

There is a growth of tissue forming around the front edges of my upper denture. It doesn't hurt, but could it be cancer?

Any unusual or unexplained growth whether in bone or in soft tissues, such as tongue, lips and cheeks, should be examined promptly by your family dentist. Although the risk of cancer is often small, the growth around your denture may need to be biopsied to identify the source.

Epulis Fissuratum

Epulis fissuratum is a type of lesion that is caused by ill fitted dentures. This can be corrected by reshaping the dentures.

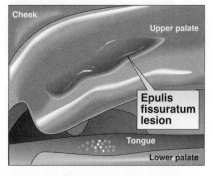

The growth of tissue around the front borders of your denture is most likely an inflammatory reaction called "epulis fissura-tum." Epulis doesn't hurt and often can go unnoticed until more extensive growth occurs. It is found most often in females and commonly affects people in their 50s.

The lesion starts near the borders of the denture that covers the gums, frequently in the front-most section.

Epulis is caused by either an ill-fitting new denture or one that has not been replaced or modified in many years. A new denture, made with overextended borders that push hard on the gums, creates an ongoing trauma. Older dentures can irritate the gums if they are not modified over time. They need to be reshaped after several years of wear to compensate for continual bone loss.

If the borders of a denture are reshaped to adapt to the mouth's floor and gums, epulis overgrowth may subside within two to three weeks. Persistent growth may require surgery. In such cases, a newly fabricated or modified denture is recommended.

Unhealed sore needs immediate attention

My father has a sore on the outside of his upper lip that hasn't healed in over two months. He refuses to have it checked since it doesn't bother him. I'm concerned for his health and would appreciate any information you can send me.

Carcinomas

Carcinomas occur when cancerous cells are present and growing in a particular area around the mouth. The example below is that of a basal cell carcinoma.

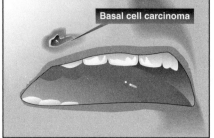

Basal cell carcinoma

The basal cell carcinoma is most common in men over 50 years of age, and occurs in areas most exposed to the sun.

Because the sore has not healed in over two months, your concern is warranted. More common ulcers, herpes and irritations of the lip usually heal within a few weeks. Persistent sores often indicate more serious and, if left untreated, deadly cancerous conditions. Your father should see a dentist or physician immediately.

Squamous cell and basal cell carcinomas are the two most likely conditions your father may have. Because of the location on the outer part of his lip or skin portion, basal cell carcinoma is more probable.

Basal cell carcinoma is the most common malignant condition of the skin. The tumor is most common in men over 50 years of age and occurs in areas most exposed to the sun. The tumor takes on many forms. Initially, it appears as a small nodule with a crusted border. Later stages appear as non-healing ulcers bordered by an elevated, darker, crusted area. Basal cell carcinoma does not appear in the oral cavity except in cases where a lesion from the skin extends into that area.

Treatment includes a biopsy to confirm and differentiate the lesion from other less common cancerous conditions. Surgical removal or radiotherapy are then recommended. Early detection and treatment reduce the possibility of complications and more extensive surgery.

Bad taste might be warning of an infection

Every once in awhile, I've noticed a bad taste in my mouth.
It goes right away, but after several days it comes back.
There's a small swelling around one of my back teeth but nothing hurts.
Now I am wondering if the swelling can be related to the bad taste?

The bad taste may be a warning sign of infection. An abscess or cyst around the gum or tooth collects pus or infectious waste products that can leak out into the mouth. In addition to the bad taste, bacteria from this location can spread to other areas, including your throat, causing infection there.

Chronic, slow, progressing infections often are not painful. The small swelling likely indicates an area of infection that needs to be promptly treated by your dentist. Even though you have no pain, an abscess can be present, causing damage to the teeth and surrounding bone. If left untreated, an infection in one area can spread to the neck and eventually cause a more serious condition. The most dangerous is cellulitis, a generalized inflammation of tissue surrounding the muscles of your mouth and neck.

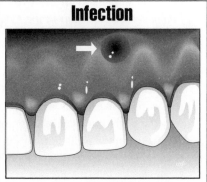

Infection

A bad taste in the mouth could be caused by an infection or abcess. Left untreated, the infection can spread to the neck or throat.

Cause of loose teeth could be an infection

I'm 78 and still have many of my front teeth, but recently they've become loose. I take good care of them, but I am concerned.

Teeth rarely loosen over a short period of time unless a severe infection is present. A slow chronic infection affects the bone and gums and teeth may loosen in the final stages.

Other causes are possible. If you do not have an appliance or restoration to replace your missing teeth, the forces of chewing will be greater on the teeth remaining, eventually weakening them. Medications can also have side effects on oral health, either making hygiene more difficult or creating an environment for bacteria that can eventually cause gum and bone disease.

Regular checkups should help ward off these problems.

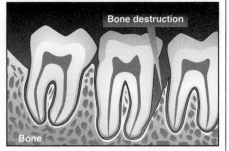

Loose Teeth

Teeth that are loose is a sign of infection in the later stages. Here is a look inside to see the result of such infection:

Bone destruction

Bone

Bone destruction is the result of unattended infection.

Dentist studies x-ray for possible abscess

*My dentist told me that he will watch one of my teeth since
he found something on the x-ray that looks like an abscess.
I've never felt any pain in the tooth, and it's otherwise normal.
Why shouldn't it be clear in the x-ray?*

There are some instances when an x-ray may have an area that appears to be an abscess on an x-ray. In such cases, your dentist uses other signs and symptoms to confirm or negate his finding. At all costs, your dentist wants to avoid treating something which may initially appear infected but requires no treatment.

Nerve entry and exit points in your jaw-bone, for example, can mimic an abscess. The most common condition is called a cementoma which, on an x-ray, resembles a tooth abscess.

Over 90 percent of cementomas are found at the base of the lower front

Cementoma

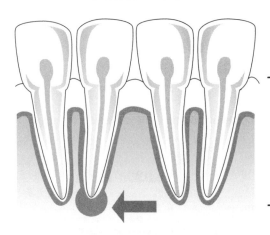

teeth. African Americans are affected more than Caucasians and Asians, and 80 percent of the lesions occur in women. They may occur on one or more teeth.

A cementoma is a swelling at the base of the front teeth. There is no clear cut reason for it, but it can grow into a more serious concern if left alone.

Often, cementomas pose no problem, and there is no associated pain or other symptom. There are no clear reasons for cementomas. Researchers believe that they are an expression of cells which make up the ligament which holds the tooth to the surrounding bone.

A cementoma can develop into a more serious condition requiring a root canal treatment, but as a general rule, if you have no discomfort, there is no need for concern. Examinations during regular checkups will show any warning signs.

Lack of saliva hinders the mouth's immunity

Our grandmother has been on medications that make her mouth very dry. Are there any precautions she needs to take for her teeth or gums?

Yes. Dry mouth is a result of reduced saliva. Saliva is linked to your body's immune system, and your grandmother's immunity to mouth diseases may be reduced.

Lack of Saliva

Dry mouth or lack of saliva can be dangerous to tooth hygiene. Saliva has agents that not only cleanse tooth surfaces, but hinder decay. Artificial lubricating agents can help dry mouth.

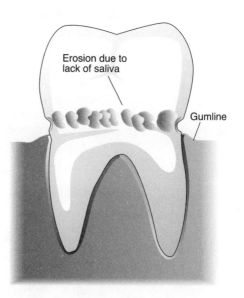

Erosion due to lack of saliva

Gumline

Saliva has many functions. Besides helping to mechanically cleanse tooth surfaces, saliva has agents that help teeth resist decay. Without the continual bathing of saliva, your grandmother's teeth will become more vulnerable to decay. Patients with dry mouth often have a dramatic increase in tooth decay. If the gums and bone have receded, exposing the roots of teeth, these may also decay.

To prevent the onset of dryness and an increased risk of cavities, your dentist may recommend these minor but effective procedures:

• Using fluoride pastes or solutions placed on the exposed roots of receding areas.
• Applying sealants to the chewing surfaces of back teeth to prevent bacteria from collecting in the small crevices of teeth.
• Suggesting artificial salivas to substitute for inadequate saliva flow or sugarless candies to help stimulate the flow of saliva.

Your dentist also may recommend dental checkups three or four times a year to closely monitor this condition.

Blue bump on the lip should be examined

I have a bluish-colored bump on my lower lip that recently appeared. It doesn't hurt. What is this and should I be concerned?

The most common lesion that fits your description is a mucocele, the result of a severed duct coming from one of the salivary glands inside your lip. Although usually blue in color, the sac may also be pinkish or yellow.

Blue Bumps

These blue bumps are caused by severed ducts from the salivary glands. Mucous collects and causes a lesion. These lesions should be removed.

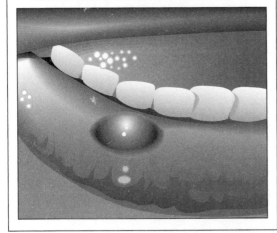

The lower lip is a common site for these lesions because this area is susceptible to trauma and has many small glands. A bump on the gums or palate is more likely caused by a more serious salivary gland tumor.

Although it doesn't hurt, you should have your dentist examine the area. Simple tests can rule out more serious conditions, such as cysts and tumors, which may be similar in appearance.

If a mucocele is not removed, mucous continues to build up, and the sac can increase in size up to a half-inch in diameter.

A larger growth that may develop on the floor of the mouth is called a ranula, from the Latin word for frog. These can grow up to two inches in diameter, often resembling a frog's belly. Like mucoceles, ranulas need to be removed.

Sunlight and stress can aggravate herpes

I get sores on my lips from herpes, especially after being out in the sun. I've tried many ointments. Is there anything new that may be better?

You may want to try creams or ointments with the compound acyclovir. Because the sore is caused by a virus, herpes simplex I, antiviral agents may be used to reduce the length or severity of these outbreaks. Treatments such as antibiotic rinses or anesthetic gels may provide some relief, but they don't attack the source of the problem.

Your sores result from a condition known as recurrent herpes labialis. There are certain physical and emotional factors that may trigger a recurrence, including sunlight, cold or stress.

The virus lives in the nerves and travels to the skin under these conditions. Limiting such sources of irritation may be your best defense. If you enjoy the sun, take added precautions to cover your lips with sunscreens to help prevent sores from forming.

Herpes Labialis

Sunlight, cold and stress are some of the factors that aggravate the recurrence of herpes labialis. The virus lives in the nerves and travels to the skin under the conditions listed above.

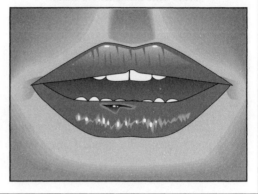

Once the sore has appeared, ointments are soothing, but the sores still may take from one to two weeks to heal. During this time, fluid from blisters may spread the virus to others, so precautions should be taken until the sores have healed.

Anesthetic or rinse relieves canker pains

I get a recurring canker sore on the inside of my upper lip.
Is there something I can do to prevent this?
Also, could you recommend the best medication for the pain?

Canker sores, or aphthous ulcers, can appear on many areas of the mouth such as the inside surface of the cheeks and lips. One can appear alone, or there may be multiple sores.

The affected region is a circular, whitish-gray ulcer usually no larger than the eraser head on a pencil and often painful. Healing occurs after one to two weeks. Depending on the degree of the condition, the sores may never reappear, or they may continue to be a problem. A few people have larger sores that may take months to heal.

Canker Pain

Canker sores have no known cause. An anesthetic gel, available at pharmacies, can offer pain relief.

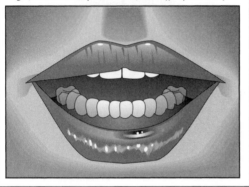

There's little you can do to prevent canker sores because their source is unknown. Studies have implicated everything from diet to bacteria to alterations in the body's immune system.

Remedies to cure the ulcers or ease the pain vary as much as the theories on their origin. Antibiotic rinses such as a tetracycline mouthwash have been used effectively. Corticosteroids in an ointment or lozenge form are also used.

Application of an anesthetic gel, available through your dentist or pharmacy, can offer pain relief while eating. For persistent outbreaks, steroids may be needed. For some people massive doses of such steroids may offer the only relief.

Stress may be factor for tongue splotches

The surface of my tongue looks splotchy like it has a rash.
My dentist assures me it's normal.
Can you tell me what causes this, and will it ever go away?

Tongue Splotches

A rash on the tongue is a condition known as migratory glossitis. It occurs without warning, and usually is not painful or harmful.

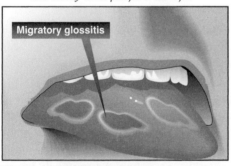

Migratory glossitis

The condition rarely goes away but is sometimes caused by some types of mouthwashes. Discontinuing mouthwash use may help the problem.

The rash on your tongue is most likely a condition known as *migratory glossitis.*

Single or multiple red areas bordered by a gray-to-white edge change position on the tongue surface. The pattern usually changes every week or month. Sometimes the same pattern will last for years. The tongue can appear normal for a time and then, without notice, the rash can appear.

It causes no problems and poses no risks for infection or

other disease. One to two percent of the population is affected. Migratory glossitis most commonly is found in young to middle-aged adults, affecting females more often.

The cause for this condition is unknown although emotional stress is an important factor that can bring on or prolong an episode.

Most rashes are not painful, but some can cause a burning sensation. In these cases, avoiding hot spicy foods and citrus fruits will lessen the burning.

Topical steroids occasionally are prescribed for relief of more serious episodes.

If you have migratory glossitis, it's unlikely it will ever go away. There can be a period of years, however, when the tongue appears normal. There is no identifiable reason for its appearance; likewise, there is no treatment for avoiding future episodes.

Some strong mouthwashes have been shown to produce this type of rash. In these rare cases, discontinuing mouthwash use will restore the tongue to normal. Occasionally these rashes indicate more severe medical disorders, which your dentist can help diagnose.

Putting out the burning tongue

I have a burning sensation on the front of my tongue.
My teeth are in good shape, and I can't think of another reason.
What causes this?

A burning sensation of the tongue can be caused by many conditions, depending on the specific location and other symptoms. Sources can range from a damaged nerve to nutritional deficiencies and blood disorders.

An irritation is the most common cause of a burning tongue. The tongue commonly develops sores near the sharp edge of a broken tooth or filling. The sores will remain aggravated until the sharp edge is smoothed out or repaired. Certain foods and

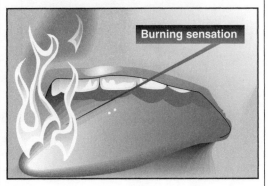

Burning Sensation

A burning sensation on the tongue can be caused by many things. Most likely it is an irritation from rough edges on teeth or nerve damage from a dental procedure.

Burning sensation

chemicals also may irritate the tongue, but pain from these sources doesn't last long.

Nerve damage incurred during dental procedures may result in a burning tongue. If an impacted wisdom tooth is near the site of the nerve that goes to the tongue, it may be damaged during extraction. One side of the tongue is affected and symptoms may last for months as the nerve heals. A small percentage of dental surgeries have this risk. Your dentist should forewarn you before surgery.

Since both sides of the front of your tongue are affected, nerve damage usually can be ruled out. A more complete medical examination may be needed after eliminating other causes.

Problems with hormone imbalance, blood disorders, gland secretion, nutritional deficiencies and allergic conditions can cause your tongue to burn.

Hairy tongue is often a symptom of illness

When I stick out my tongue, I can see a brownish hair-like growth on my tongue that covers the surface. It almost looks dirty, but I can't clean it off. What is it, and how can I get rid of it?

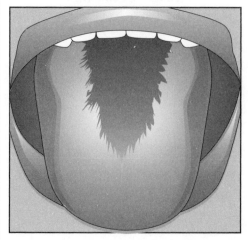

Hairy Tongue

Hairy tongue can be attributed to drugs or poor oral hygiene. Tongue brushing techniques can help this condition.

"Hairy tongue" develops from changes in the cells of your tongue's surface. They become longer after retaining abnormal amounts of keratin which are normally sloughed off. When noticed for the first time, the length and number of hair-like filaments can be alarming. However, there is often no reason for concern.

Investigators think several factors may prompt this condition. Tobacco use, antibiotics and oral medications, infections and poor oral hygiene are all thought to be related to, if not directly a cause of, hairy tongue.

The condition is seen most often in people with serious diseases such as cancerous tumors and AIDS.

Hairy tongue is treated by improving tongue brushing techniques and cutting the elongated filaments. The color of these filaments may vary from white to tan to black. Chemicals and food stains are thought to cause the variation. All forms, regardless of color and degree, are treated the same. Even with successful treatment, however, the filaments can persist and may change color.

Bony growths in jaw seldom need removal

I have these bony lumps on the inside of my lower jaw. They don't hurt and my last dentist said they were normal. How or why did they form?

The overgrowth of bone you describe are called "*tori.*" They can appear on either the upper or lower jaw, growing slowly by age 30. Tori usually form on both sides and grow from the base of the teeth just below the gumline. They may appear as small bumps or extend laterally along or under the tongue. You are among the estimated 12 percent of adults that have these growths.

Tori are found in the middle of the palate in about 30 percent of adults. Females and ethnic

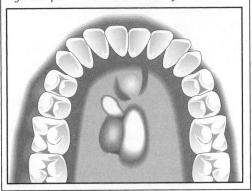

Bony Growths

Bony growths under the tongue that sprout from the lower jaw called "tori" are common in adults. These growths pose no threat and are usually not removed.

groups such as African Americans and Eskimos are more likely to develop tori.

Less common are *exostoses*, bony overgrowths under the gums on the outside of the upper or lower jaw. Although they seldom must be removed, tori or exostoses should be examined by a dentist. They should be distinguished from other bone disorders which may require surgical removal. There are certain situations when tori are surgically removed to eliminate obstruction and irritation for those wearing dentures.

Tori may get in the way during certain dental procedures, such as the taking of x-rays or dental impressions.

Tori are believed to be hereditary and an evolutionary answer to a reinforced jaw or chewing strength. Some investigators believe exostoses are formed in response to extreme biting stress.

Smooth surfaces take the bite out of fibromas

Sometimes during a meal, I accidentally bite my cheek.
There's a small lump that has developed that won't go away.
Is there anything I can do to get rid of it?

Cheek Biting

Rough areas on teeth, irritation from braces, or cheek biting can be the cause of fibromas. These lesions can be surgically removed by your dentist.

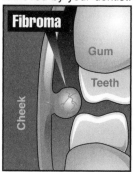

Fibroma

Gum

Teeth

Cheek

Ongoing irritation or trauma from biting any part of your mouth can turn into a persistent sore or lump. The lump is most likely a fibroma, a non-cancerous irritation of tissue that can be easily removed. Until the source of the irritation is removed, the lump will likely remain.

The causes of irritation are numerous and may involve a single tooth or group of teeth. Broken or cracked teeth, especially those with sharp edges, can irritate your tongue or cheek. Certain dental appliances, including orthodontic brackets and partial denture clasps and attachments, can also aggravate areas of your mouth.

There are causes of trauma that may occur over years for no apparent reason. For example, when extensive restorations have been completed on back teeth, either with crowns, bridges or partial dentures, the position of teeth is important. In addition to their function of chewing, these teeth support the cheek as you close your mouth. If they are not in a specific position, the cheek may be more likely to get trapped in between the teeth when you close them together.

Although the fibroma may reoccur with continued irritation, the cheek usually heals quickly with no adverse signs. Your dentist may have the tissue biopsied to detect any remote chance of cancer.

Removing the source of trauma can be either simple or complicated. In the case of a single tooth with broken or sharp edges, a simple procedure of smoothing down the edge or covering the affected area with a filling can solve the problem.

For minor sores from orthodontic brackets or metal attachments on partial dentures, a piece of soft dental wax can be molded over the tooth area until the sore is healed. In instances where considerable restorations have been done, the contour and position of some teeth may need to be altered to avoid continual cheek biting. More difficult cases may involve remaking part or all of an appliance to adequately support the cheek.

Each case is individual in its needs and sensitivity to treatment. Constant communication between you and your dentist will help find the cause and best treatment.

Hepatitis B virus is carried after recovery

About five years ago, I had hepatitis. Recently, my dentist asked me to check with my physician to see if I might still be a carrier. He said I could still spread the disease. Is this possible?

If you have had hepatitis B or "serum hepatitis," you may be a carrier. More than 300,000 new carriers of this form of hepatitis are diagnosed each year.

There are several types of hepatitis, but the two most common are hepatitis A, known as "infectious hepatitis," and hepatitis B. If your physician or dentist classifies your disease as type A, there is almost no chance of carrying the virus after the disease has run its course. However, as many as 20 percent of those with hepatitis B continue to carry the virus.

If you have never been tested for the possibility of being a carrier, you may unnecessarily be placing others at risk. You should consider getting an examination. If you are identified as a carrier, your dentist may choose to take additional precautions. Although a vaccine for hepatitis B became available in 1982, some health care professionals have never been vaccinated.

Drugs can suppress facial nerve pains

I've just been diagnosed with trigeminal neuralgia and am confused about what can be done to correct it. Will the sharp pains subside?

Trigeminal neuralgia is a painful condition that affects the facial nerves associated with the trigeminal nerve. This nerve has branches that extend from the base of the eye to the mouth. People affected complain of extreme episodes of pain that are "stabbing," "burning" or "shocking." Episodes can last seconds or a few minutes and can go into remission as suddenly as they appear. Trigeminal neuralgia is more frequently found in women and in people over 60 years old.

There is no known cause, although many theories suggest various possibilities. Therefore, treatment can often only diminish the symptoms. Anti-seizure drugs are often prescribed to suppress the pain. More severe cases are treated with surgical procedures that can possibly alleviate the condition. In many instances, however, the results of such procedures can be unpredictable.

The remissions with no associated pain can last weeks or several months, which may influence the decision to try a more permanent treatment. Otherwise, drugs and other forms of care are more common methods to help cope with the pain.

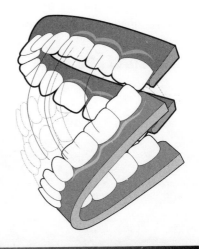

Chapter 15

Bite and
Jaw Joint Problems

Abrasion can cause grooves near gumline

I have grooves in my teeth that are near the gumline.
Some of the deeper ones are sensitive when I drink something cold.
What causes these and how are they treated?

Cervical Erosions

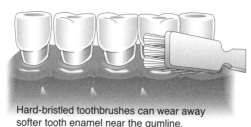

Hard-bristled toothbrushes can wear away softer tooth enamel near the gumline.

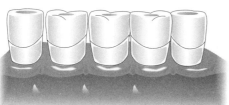

Fillings and bonding can repair damage done by the toothbrush and abrasive toothpastes.

Grooves in your teeth often are caused by abrasion. Brushing teeth forcefully or with a hard-bristled brush can wear away teeth. The gumline portion is affected first since the outer hard enamel layer is thinnest in this area. The underlying dentin layer is softer and will wear away faster. Abrasive toothpastes also can increase the risk of developing these grooves. Biting problems are another source of tooth grooves. Researchers report that undue stress placed on certain teeth can cause these grooves to develop.

If the grooves are noticeably deep, a tooth-colored composite filling usually can protect and restore a tooth. Sensitivity to cold and air is a first sign that such a procedure may be needed.

Recession of the gums is commonly found at or near the groove areas. Newly exposed root surfaces of a tooth may also be sensitive and require additional treatment.

Preventing further wear is the ultimate goal in treating such a problem. Hard-bristled toothbrushes should be replaced with soft ones. Forceful brushing back and forth across the gumline of teeth should be corrected. When tooth grooves are accompanied by gum recession, brushing should be done in small circular motions with the toothbrush bristles at a 45-degree angle to the gumline. The brush handle then should be turned and carried downward. Use of abrasive toothpastes should also be discontinued.

If biting problems are the cause, tooth adjustments should be made. In a normal, healthy condition, teeth make contact evenly and at the same time.

If left untreated or if the abrasion continues, the groove depth can reach the nerve of a tooth. At this point, root canal treatment may be needed.

Adjustments can help take a bite out of grind

I've had pain in my jaw joint for several years and recently a dentist suggested that my bite needs adjusting. How can he be sure this is the cause and are there any problems with doing the procedure?

Pain in the jaw joint can stem from many causes. Bite problems commonly are associated with joint pain.

Several clues help your dentist in determining the relationship between a poor bite and joint discomfort. Areas of advanced tooth wear may indicate habits like teeth clenching and grinding or teeth that are positioned out of alignment. If grinding alone is the cause of tooth wear, then a protective plastic appliance can be made to protect the teeth. However, if the alignment of teeth is slightly off and if the grinding is merely a symptom of this misalignment, then adjusting the bite may be needed.

There are varying degrees of bite adjustment depending on the severity of poorly aligned teeth.

Jaw Pain

Sometimes jaw pain can be caused by the misalignment of the bite. This can be remedied by the shaping of teeth with a high-speed drill.

Back teeth

Drill to shape teeth

Corrected bite

When the biting surfaces vary only slightly from an ideal position, a process called selective grinding is usually recommended. Your dentist grinds away small selective areas of the outer enamel biting surfaces of the teeth. Slight discrepancies in the way teeth contact each other can cause significant pain in the jaw joint. Should there be greater discrepancies in the way the teeth meet, orthodontic movement or fillings may be needed.

When your teeth come together in such a way that they do not contact each other evenly, there may be stress to the individual teeth and/or the jaw joint. Likewise, if your jaw joint closes in a way that differs from the position in which your teeth should come together, this difference can result in joint pain. Efforts to correct or adjust your bite allow both your teeth and your jaw joint to close together in a comfortable manner.

Tooth grinding cause difficult to pinpoint

My husband grinds his teeth at night making a loud noise.
Can you tell me if this causes tooth damage and how to stop this habit?

Bruxism Solution

Grinding teeth can wear them down. Sometimes into the nerve, which can be painful. This is one solution.

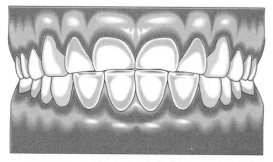

Worn teeth due to bruxism

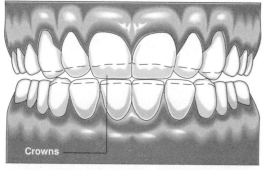

Crowns

A removable plastic bite appliance is made for the patient to slow the grinding of the teeth. After three months of wearing, the appliance crowns are added.

Tooth grinding or bruxism is the excessive wear of tooth surfaces caused by grating lower teeth against upper teeth. Prolonged bruxism can expose the tooth's nerve, causing pain. This may occur in people of any age and often continues for years.

Although usually occurring during sleep, grinding may also occur during the day. In addition to the wearing away of teeth and added stress to fillings in the area, your bite and jaw joint are also affected. Bruxism frequently causes muscle and joint pain.

To stop the grinding both you and your dentist need to search for the underlying source of the problem. Changes in your bite may be a cause. Factors such as tooth loss or changes in the position of your teeth can start bruxism. Stress, although a contributing and possible causing factor, is all-too-often mistakenly named as the cause.

What can be done to correct the problem? Sometimes a simple adjustment helping the teeth to meet more evenly can be the answer. Many times, however, the source is not found or is too complex to easily correct. As a preliminary treatment, your dentist will usually make a mouthguard or bite splint to prevent further tooth wear.

Untreated tooth wear can cause problems

The edges of my front two teeth are rough and jagged.
They don't hurt, but I'm worried they may continue to wear away.
Do I need to have anything done to them?

There are several causes for the biting edges of your front teeth to become worn and jagged. Accidents and traumatic injuries can chip and fracture small pieces of your teeth. Acidic fruit juices and soda eroding the outside surfaces and stomach acids wearing away the inside surfaces can thin the edges of front teeth. Continual and unnatural wear of teeth in one jaw contacting the teeth in the other can wear and fracture the edges.

Initially, the treatment of the problem may involve smoothing of a weakened edge. For more severe cases, a tooth-colored composite material or porcelain crown or covering may be needed.

If acids, either from foods or the stomach (in people suffering from ulcer conditions) are the cause of the tooth wear, the mouth contents need to be neutralized. A paste of baking soda and water should be swished for 30 seconds, to allow contact with the teeth. Tooth brushing should be done only after this neutralization is complete. Unnatural tooth wear may need to be corrected by adjustments. Removal of jagged edges on contact areas may provide treatment for minor cases.

Continual wear can leave teeth prone to more severe breaks, exposure of nerves, and in some cases, tooth loss.

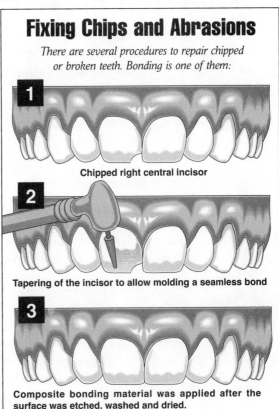

Fixing Chips and Abrasions

There are several procedures to repair chipped or broken teeth. Bonding is one of them:

1

Chipped right central incisor

2

Tapering of the incisor to allow molding a seamless bond

3

Composite bonding material was applied after the surface was etched, washed and dried.

Cracked tooth can cause sporadic pain

Every once in a while when I'm chewing, I have a sharp pain.
It goes away quickly, and it may not come back for several weeks.
Nothing else bothers the tooth. I haven't seen a dentist since
the discomfort is so infrequent. Should I be concerned?

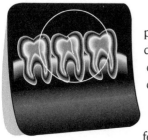

If your tooth occasionally is sensitive to biting pressure, it may have a crack, a condition that may be difficult to diagnose. However, you should alert your dentist of the sensitivity. There are tests that can help detect a cracked tooth.

Cracks are defects that usually develop as a result of biting trauma. People who chew ice, nuts or firm foods are more prone to cracks. Other dental procedures such as a root canal may also dry out the tooth structure, making it more prone to cracking.

Initially, cracks are hard to detect since they may not be visible on x-rays. Telling your dentist is important because observing your symptoms may catch the problem early. If left untreated, the crack may become more extensive and difficult to treat.

Treatment involves placing a crown or cap around the crack. If the crack extends near or into the root, a root canal may be needed.

Study of dental history takes bite out of plight

Every now and then, while I am eating, I suddenly bite
the side of my inner cheek. What causes me to bite myself?
Is it because I have too much flab in my cheeks?
What can I do to eliminate this nuisance?

Cheek biting occurs when the tissue of your cheek folds inward as your jaw closes and gets trapped between your teeth. Normally, the outer contour of your upper teeth keeps the tissue from getting caught. Misaligned teeth, improper tooth contour, broken or unrestored teeth and new prosthetic appliances are among the problems that cause cheek biting. For people with thick or heavy tissue on the inside of their cheek, such a problem may be more prevalent.

The ability of your dentist to identify and treat the source of your problem depends on knowing the onset and frequency of it. For example, did the problem start after a new cap or bridge was placed or after losing or not repairing a broken-down back tooth? If the signs of cheek biting start suddenly, there usually is an identifiable cause that can be easily treated.

If, however, the problem has existed for years and is now becoming more of a nuisance, then treatment may be more extensive. Treatment may be as simple as rounding off the outside contour of a single tooth. More involved treatment may include orthodontics, restorative work or alterations in an existing partial or complete denture if such appliances are being worn.

Tooth buildup okay if length's involved

My lower front teeth look short from the constant wear of biting. They are only sensitive when I have cold foods or fruit juices. Should these be repaired, and can they be made longer again?

Although it is common for tooth wear to occur over time, some people have more dramatic loss, requiring restoration. Tooth wear can occur in many locations on a tooth's surface and is common on the biting edges of your lower front teeth.

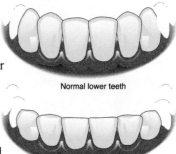

Normal lower teeth

If your teeth are sensitive only to acidic fruits, a simple coating may be applied to alleviate this discomfort. Small defects or pits in the biting edges can additionally be repaired with tooth-colored composite fillings.

Worn lower teeth

Although it is often possible to restore some of the original length of a worn tooth, it may not be desirable. Worn teeth are usually caused by gradual abrasion against upper teeth. If the length is restored, it must be done in such a way as to not interfere or contact heavily with opposing teeth when you bite and chew. Regaining the length of your lower teeth may look aesthetically unnatural if surrounding teeth have been worn down.

If there is only slight discomfort and minimal concern for appearance, conservative treatment with little or no restoration is sufficient. Moderate pain or severe loss of tooth structure may require more extensive buildup or crowns to protect and reposition teeth. Surrounding teeth may also need to be restored, both functionally and aesthetically.

Overbite trauma goes beyond cosmetics

My dentist told me I have a deep overbite. Other than appearance are there any problems I may develop because of it?

Overbite is defined by the distance the upper teeth close vertically past the lower teeth when the jaw is closed. That distance is often only a few millimeters, but in some cases the overlap is so extreme that the upper teeth cover the lower ones. Problems with a deep overbite are related to the degree of the overbite and how well you are adapting to the way your teeth are positioned.

Overbites

An Overbite is how much overlap the teeth have.

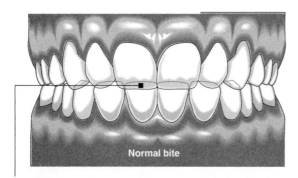

Normal bite

Lower teeth behind upper

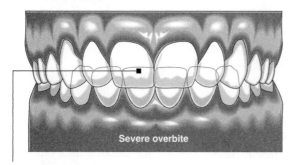

Severe overbite

Lower teeth behind upper

Deep overbites can cause many dental problems including excessive wear of teeth, trauma to the surrounding gums, and jaw joint problems. Potential problems can be detected during a dental exam. If your jaw and teeth are unable to adapt to a deep overbite, you may suffer swollen gums, accelerated wear or chipping of teeth, pain during or after meals and difficulty biting into foods.

Minimal problems may be corrected with plastic mouth guards worn over the teeth or by removing small areas of the teeth obstructing normal jaw movement.

In some cases, the lower jaw cannot move forward, which restricts movement during chewing. Serious conditions such as these may have to be corrected by an orthodontic specialist who can change the position of the teeth by fitting braces. Jaw surgery may be recommended in cases where orthodontics are not enough.

If you're experiencing jaw or chewing discomfort, inform your dentist. Waiting may make the condition more difficult to treat.

Clicking sound while chewing is common

My jaw makes a clicking sound when I'm chewing something hard.
Nothing hurts, but I've read that this can be associated with joint
problems. Is that true, and if so, what can be done about it?

Joint sounds are common during chew-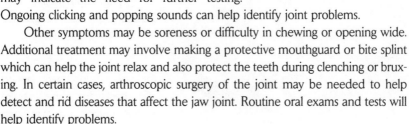
ing and do not necessarily indicate a dys-
function or abnormality in the jaw joint. As
many as three-quarters of the population
has some form of detectable joint sound.

During routine oral examinations, your
dentist might place a finger over the joint
while you open and close. This technique
helps detect more prominent sounds that
may indicate the need for further testing.
Ongoing clicking and popping sounds can help identify joint problems.

Other symptoms may be soreness or difficulty in chewing or opening wide.
Additional treatment may involve making a protective mouthguard or bite splint
which can help the joint relax and also protect the teeth during clenching or brux-
ing. In certain cases, arthroscopic surgery of the joint may be needed to help
detect and rid diseases that affect the jaw joint. Routine oral exams and tests will
help identify problems.

Jaw aches connected to hunched posture

My sister complains about headaches and jaw aches. Her posture
is bad (she hunches over), and our dentist says this may be the cause.
He made her a special mouthguard that helps.
Can you explain what it does?

Posture has long been associated with headaches and backaches. Poor posture may put your spine in a position which may cause stress to the jaw joint.

Your jaw can close in two different ways. The first is determined by how
the upper and lower teeth meet. Jaw muscles also play a role in guiding the
joint. When they are relaxed, your jaws can close in another position. Although
the final closing position of your jaws may be the same under both conditions,
often they are quite different. Your muscles may need to work in moving your
jaws to a position where the teeth can meet.

Since your sister hunches over, her lower jaw has a tendency to move forward. In addition, her skull will move back on top of the highest bone of the spinal column. Both movements can cause stress on the joints, bones and muscles.

Hunch Pain

Some bodies are able to adapt to changes in posture. But for those that can't, the stress may result in headaches.

The normal posture position centers jaw joints and muscles.

Bad posture can sometimes cause jaw misalignment, putting stress on the muscles, joints and spine.

Normal Posture

Tilting your head back too far causes your lower jaw to slide backward. When you're getting a filling, a dentist often will place you upright to see how your teeth meet. Your bite may feel okay when lying down, yet needs adjustment in an upright position.

The special mouthguard that your dentist makes is called an anterior repositioning splint. It helps teeth align in a position that reduces muscle strain caused by an awkward posture.

A bad slouching posture causes the jaw to jut forward and stresses the muscles and joint. The spine is also strained causing headache pain.

Bad Posture

Stress causes a real pain in the jaw and neck

Our family dentist is treating my wife for a dental condition called myofacial pain dysfunction. What is it and what causes it?

Myofacial pain dysfunction refers to several symptoms involving the limited movement of the lower jaw, or mandible. Seventy percent of the patients have headaches or pain in their jaw joints. For 28 percent of them, facial and neck pain is the second most common complaint. Other symptoms include ear pain or ringing in the ear, nausea, tension, fatigue and loss of balance.

The pain can be episodic or chronic, mild or severe. The ear and the area just in front of it are usually affected, although the sensations may spread throughout the face.

Studies indicate many factors, physiological and psychological, may play a role: low self-esteem, perfectionism, self-criticism, stress, even teeth grinding.

Myofacial pain dysfunction affects about 88 percent of the population; only a few seek treatment. Your dentist can help you sort through these possibilities.

Music-playing fiddles with teeth alignment

I've been playing the violin professionally for many years. Recently, my jaw has begun to ache on the same side that I rest my violin. Can my playing cause the jaw pain, and what can I do to stop the ache?

A current Gallup Poll estimates that there are 1.79 million string instrumentalists in the United States. They use varying biting relationships, and their lower jaw helps brace the instrument on their shoulder. Many of these players experience fatigue and pain in their jaws or neck and shoulders. Additional strain may occur when the head bobs while playing.

Temporomandibular joint or TMJ pain can sometimes be relieved by resting the instrument on the clavicle shelf rather than on the shoulder. Other dental appliances like a dental splint worn over the biting surfaces of the teeth may help.

There are additional dental problems that musicians may face. Approximately 1.86 million wind instrumentalists use their teeth, tongue and lips in myriad ways to play their instruments.

Problems vary from gum disease to tooth movement as a result of pressure against a mouthpiece or from tongue thrusting. As these musicians develop a playing embouchure, their tooth biting relationship changes.

To correct the changes and prevent further problems, treatment involving dental appliances may be necessary. For example, players needing to close over a wedge-shaped mouthpiece may wear an orthodontic appliance that will stabilize the teeth braced against it.

Since there are numerous dental problems that can be caused by different instruments, consult your dentist regarding an appropriate treatment specific to your problem.

Chewing over mom's jaw joint arthroscopy

My mother has difficulty eating since her jaw gets so sore.
An oral surgeon has recommended a procedure called arthroscopy.
Can her condition be cured without surgery?

Arthroscopy

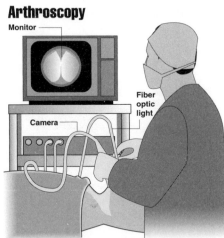

Arthroscopy uses a tiny video camera to view the workings of a joint. This enables the surgeon to see the joint and treat it without a large incision.

Arthroscopy is a surgical method of viewing and performing jaw joint surgery within the confines of the joint spaces. Cutting adhesions which limit the motion of the joint, and draining fluids from—and injecting medicines into—diseased areas are just some of the uses of such surgery.

Three instruments are used in arthroscopy. The first is a telescope, a thin tube with internal lenses that is used to magnify or view the joint and its surroundings. Another instrument is used for penetrating the joint and for surgical procedures which are performed once inside the joint area. A fiber optic light is the last tool which illuminates the area being examined.

Pain in the joint or limitations when talking and eating can sometimes be relieved with other devices and non-surgical treatments. Joint surgery is recommended only when non-surgical methods fail.

Most oral surgeons are well-qualified in arthroscopic procedures. Since the recommendation has already been made to your mother, other non-surgical techniques have likely failed. The procedure is safe, effective and useful in improving many joint disorders. Even with successful surgery, however, follow-up exercises and continued treatment need to be followed diligently.

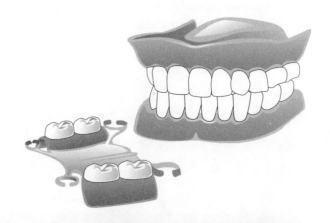

Chapter 16

Partial and
Full Dentures

Removable Prosthodontics
- Prostho (prosthesis)
- removable appliance to restore teeth

Gold is more pliable, reliable for partials

My dentist recommended a gold partial denture for my lower jaw.
Some friends of mine had silver-colored chrome ones made.
Why has gold been chosen in my case, especially
since the gold partial costs more?

Dentist

The most common metal used in partial dentures is a chromium cobalt alloy. Factors such as strength, light weight, good adaptable fit and low cost make it attractive for many patients' needs.

Gold alloys are also used and are useful in making partials for several reasons. In cases where there are many clasps and attachments requiring an accurate fit, gold is more reliable and predictable. Although the cast gold partial is not as strong as cast chromium cobalt, it is pliable. Such an advantage is useful for distributing stress from clasps and attachments to the teeth. Finally, a gold alloy partial may be a good link with the gold fillings frequently used to restore teeth to which a partial attaches. Some patients experience a minor shock or metallic taste when dissimilar metals are used and are in direct contact. Gold is less likely to produce such a reaction.

Less bulky partial fittings cost more

My new partial denture attaches to almost every tooth in my lower jaw.
It seems there is a lot of unnecessary metal there.
Can it be made to anchor to just a few of my teeth?

The metal attachments on partial dentures function to keep the denture stable. Appliances like partials can rock side to side and front to back. Metal attachments to the teeth keep the denture fixed during eating and talking. They are constructed to distribute the stress from such functions over the remaining teeth and bone. Clasps and attachments also serve to retain the appliance so that it fits snugly in the jaw and yet can be easily removed.

If you are concerned with the number and bulk of attachments, let your dentist know. Several types of special customized fittings can be incorporated into the construction of the partial denture. They may not be routinely recommended because there is often an additional expense. First time partial denture wearers should spend considerable time with their dentist discussing the different methods of constructing their appliance. Those replacing an existing partial may want to express concerns about their old partial to avoid continuing problems.

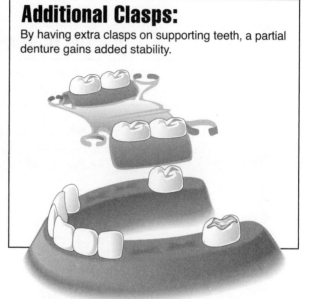

Additional Clasps:

By having extra clasps on supporting teeth, a partial denture gains added stability.

Breakage is not always the end for partial denture

One of the metal clasps on my partial denture broke recently, and now the partial rocks from side to side. Can this be repaired?

Metal clasps on a partial denture function to stabilize the device by wrapping around some of your natural teeth. Clasps may break off due to biting stress. If a clasp breaks, the denture is more likely to move since it is less stable.

There are three solutions to this problem. The first is to re-solder the metal clasp to the metal framework of the partial denture. To do this, acrylic teeth and artificial gums need to be removed and reset after the attachment is made.

A soldered clasp is often not as strong as the original casting, so minor modifications must be made to help guarantee the same break will not occur again. In some cases it is impossible to solder a clasp, so other options must be explored.

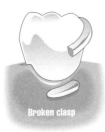

Broken clasp

A second solution is to use wire clasps that can attach to the acrylic portion of a partial denture. Although not as strong as cast metal clasps, they provide some comfort and stabilization.

Partial Denture Breaks

Partial denture clasps that break can be soldered back together, but the clasp will not be as strong as the original.

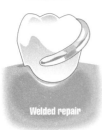

Welded repair

The last possibility is to remake and redesign a partial denture. Although more costly, this provides the most long-lasting result.

Material of plates is based on needs

Why are some partial dental plates made of plastic while others are made of metal? Which is better and why?

Materials and design of partial dentures vary considerably with each person. Different variables, such as the number of teeth and the health of the gums and bone surrounding them, must be considered. Partial dentures can be made of plastic, metal or a combination of both. The plastic used primarily is acrylic while metals can vary from chromium to gold alloys.

Part of material selection is based on future needs. In general, plastic is used in areas that may undergo change. Areas of bone resorption or surrounding teeth that are compromised and have questionable outcomes are factors that are also considered. Adding additional artificial teeth or other areas of acrylic can easily be done to an existing acrylic partial denture. Transitional or temporary partial dentures often are made of acrylic to accommodate these changing needs.

Metal and plastic partials are a combination of strength (metal) and versatility (plastic).

Metals are used because a thinner and less bulky plate can be made while still maintaining strength. The choice of metals can vary from chromium alloys that are more stiff to gold alloys that provide more flexibility, especially in areas that hold or surround existing teeth. Often, a more precise fit can be achieved using gold alloys. Your dentist will select the material or combination of materials based on the individual needs of your teeth and the surrounding gums and bone.

Fit of partial denture is subject to shifting

My partial denture rocks back and forth. I haven't had any discomfort for years but am wondering why has it started to move?

There are many causes for a rocking movement with partial dentures. Decreasing bone support and tooth movement both may be playing a role in your discomfort.

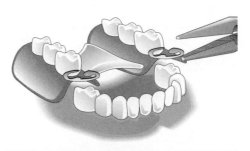

Partial dentures usually are constructed of metal and acrylic. They replace missing teeth and stabilize the remaining teeth. The appliance distributes chewing forces evenly over a broad area, including those areas where teeth have been extracted. Since bone and teeth change with the constant stress of chewing, the fit of the partial may be altered over time.

Loose partials are caused by many factors. Bone changes or teeth moving can be some causes. It is important to keep partials adjusted in order to distribute chewing pressures.

Commonly, your jaw bone recedes so that an area of support can no longer function. If this is the case, your partial needs to be adjusted. Usually, acrylic is added to compensate for bone loss.

If tooth movement or support is the cause of rocking, tightening the metal clasp which is attached to the tooth or replacing or adding a new clasp may solve the problem.

If you notice any changes in the stability of your partial denture, you should visit your dentist immediately. Waiting can cause low grade trauma to remaining teeth, which stabilize the partial. These supporting teeth can then become loose and be prematurely lost.

A partial may require other tooth repairs

To replace some of my missing teeth, I am having a partial denture made. The dentist wants to first replace several of my amalgam fillings with gold ones. He claims that these will last longer and help support the partial denture more. My silver ones have been doing fine for years. Why not just leave them alone?

All teeth and existing restorations should be examined when making a partial denture. Areas of decay should be restored first. Fillings that are either worn, broken or too large to withstand the forces of a partial denture should then be restored.

As a general rule, large silver fillings in teeth that will help support and stabilize the partial denture should be replaced by cast gold fillings or crowns. The added stress from clasps and fittings on the denture to the fillings is enough to cause them to break down and fracture. Replacing a filling or fixing a tooth fracture after a partial has been made is more complicated.

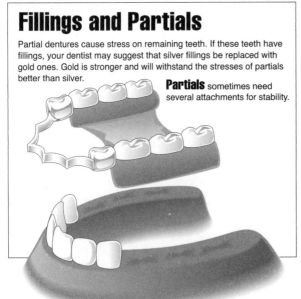

Fillings and Partials

Partial dentures cause stress on remaining teeth. If these teeth have fillings, your dentist may suggest that silver fillings be replaced with gold ones. Gold is stronger and will withstand the stresses of partials better than silver.

Partials sometimes need several attachments for stability.

Before making a new partial denture, new fillings are also made which correct the alignment of teeth. In some cases, a more upright or ideal position of a tooth is needed before constructing the partial denture.

If you follow these recommendations from your dentist, your final denture will function better, and last longer.

Biting your cheek may be a partial problem

While wearing my new lower partial denture, I began biting my cheek when chewing food. Will my dentist be able to correct this?

I am assuming you are wearing a lower partial denture because you have lost several of your lower teeth. The resulting facial changes may be causing your problem.

When back teeth are lost and go unreplaced for several years, the bite changes, corners of the lips may fold inward, and facial muscles surrounding the mouth may lose their tone.

A lower denture is meant to simulate exactly the position of your original teeth. That position usually helps keep the cheek from being trapped between your teeth as did your natural teeth before they were lost. Cheek biting may indicate that the position of the teeth needs to be changed.

But try wearing the partial denture for several weeks; you may just need to get used to it. If the problem persists, see your dentist.

If your denture replaced a worn but well-made denture that didn't cause cheek-biting, alterations may be minor. People who go several years without restoring missing teeth have a more difficult time adjusting.

Cheek Biting

Missing teeth should be corrected by replacement. Cheek biting may occur once partials are added if teeth are missing for an extended amount of time.

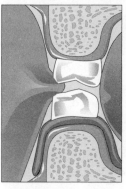

Cheek biting by partials can be caused by the facial changes due to missing teeth for an extended amount of time.

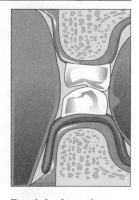

Partial alterations can aleviate this problem.

If alterations don't help, your upper teeth may need to be modified. Changing their outer contour can keep the inside of your cheek from being caught.

Anchors for dentures get to root of problem

I have the roots of two teeth left in my lower jaw.
My dentist wants to make a denture that fits over them.
Wouldn't it just be easier to have them removed?

Retaining the roots of your teeth has advantages. If the roots are strong enough and in a useful location, they may help to anchor a denture that fits over them.

Protective coatings can be made to cover the roots and keep them from decaying. These roots can then help to hold a denture in place. Fittings can also

Dentures with Roots

Leaving tooth roots in the mouth help anchor dentures by use of posts or connecting bars.

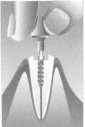 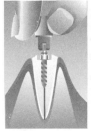 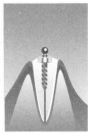

The root canal bored out with a finger wrench.

A post is screwed into the space.

The post is cemented and is topped with a mounting head for the denture connector.

be made for the roots which interlock with attachments placed in the denture. There are many other types of fittings which provide varying degrees of support.

For example, sometimes a horizontal bar can be constructed which attaches two or more roots. Clips then positioned in the denture can attach to the fixed bar.

Keeping healthy roots helps to maintain the bone surrounding them. Over a period of years, bone recession often accompanies the wearing of a denture. Retaining the roots of teeth helps the bone surrounding them resist this gradual recession.

Extracting teeth is simple and often less costly than procedures needed to retain them. However, important benefits are lost after tooth extraction. Besides providing anchors to stabilize a denture, removing teeth will also cause an increase in bone loss.

Transitional denture allows for change

After losing some of my teeth, my dentist recommended that I have a lower partial denture made. She wants to make a temporary one first, and after several months a permanent one. Is this necessary? Why can't she wait until the gums heal, then make the final denture?

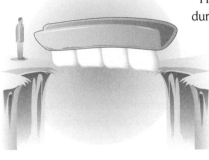

Having two dentures made at different times during your treatment has many benefits.

A temporary partial denture or "transitional partial" allows your dentist additional time to determine factors that will influence the final design of a permanent partial denture. Because several of your teeth were recently removed, the healing of these areas is one such factor.

Gum disease and tooth problems may add additional uncertainty to the eventual number of remaining teeth. Treating the gum disease and repairing the tooth problems may be a slow process with an unpredictable outcome.

A final partial is based on a design that will withstand the daily stresses of chewing and talking. The denture must also be adaptable to function when problems arise later, such as when there is an additional loss of teeth and bone support. The original partial design can still be modified and used.

When there are too many factors that remain uncertain, your dentist will construct a transitional partial which can easily adapt to these changes. Any additional cost or discomfort from wearing a transitional partial will far outweigh the costs and pain from a permanent design that will not adapt to changes in your mouth.

There are many points to chew in selecting dentures

Our dentist asked my father for an old photograph
when he made a set of dentures for him. Can a dentist
tell what the teeth should look like without a photograph?

Your dentist has been complete and careful in selecting teeth that will look natural. An old photograph may give him a better idea of the form of your father's original teeth. As there are hundreds of shapes, sizes and colors, several tooth types may be appropriate, but only one is unique.

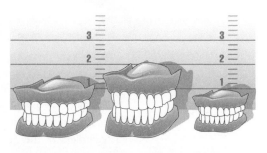

In general, the shape of teeth is related to the shape of the face. The size, although usually proportional to face size, is variable. The color of teeth also varies. Without remaining teeth to compare, a photograph may be the next best thing.

Without these aids your dentist will base the selection of teeth on facial shape, size of the mouth, skin tone and age.

Alignment of the teeth is another important consideration. Deliberate effort is often made to place the teeth slightly out of position since a perfect row can look too artificial. Individual characteristics of teeth such as spaces and slight protrusions can help give a more natural appearance.

Many factors are considered when choosing and setting the teeth for dentures. Unless all are taken into account, the result may not look natural.

Tools make a clean sweep of dentures

Every time we eat meat, my father traps some on his partial plate and in between some of his teeth. Is there an easy way to clean a partial? Can it be made so it doesn't trap food as much?

Partial dentures often trap food particles. Metal clasps around your teeth that hold the denture in place may catch food strands, and spaces between a partial plate and teeth can trap food debris. Food also can get lodged underneath the sections of a partial denture that rest on the gums.

Denture Cleaning

There are several forms of denture cleansing, here are a few techniques:

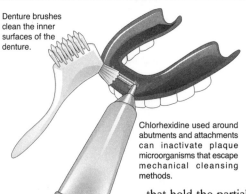

Denture brushes clean the inner surfaces of the denture.

Chlorhexidine used around abutments and attachments can inactivate plaque microorganisms that escape mechanical cleansing methods.

There are many designs of partial dentures that can restore any given mouth. If one design becomes uncomfortable and difficult to use, your dentist may propose another type of construction. It is hard to predict how well any individual will tolerate a given partial design. There are, however, certain types of partials that generally provide added comfort and stability, and which are less likely to trap food. Precision partials, for example, utilize interlocking attachments that hold the partial to your teeth. These substitute for the more traditional clasps that wrap around certain teeth.

Regardless of the design, there will often be awkward spaces that require special cleaning accessories to help keep food and plaque from building up around your teeth and the partial denture. Interdental brushes help clean wide spaces underneath bars and other metal attachments that link certain teeth. They have a small brush head with bristles that are longer than a traditional toothbrush bristle for easier access to these spaces.

Denture brushes are larger and help clean a denture after it has been removed from the mouth. They come in a wide variety of shapes and sizes to fit your individual needs. Specially shaped toothpicks can also provide a way to clean difficult to reach areas. Finally, there are brushlike flosses called "dental yarn" or "super floss" which help clean wide spaces between teeth and attachment points between a partial denture and your natural teeth.

Your dentist will provide options to make any adjustment to a new partial denture easier. He or she may also suggest some additional cleaning tools to help clean your partial and your remaining, teeth. Good oral hygiene is the most important aspect of retaining any dental restoration.

Cheap dentures may cost more in long run

How much does cost influence the quality of dentures?

If you find someone to make you an "inexpensive set" of dentures, you just may be looking again within a few years. The price for a set of upper and lower dentures varies, depending upon individual needs. Several visits are required to ensure a functional, comfortable and aesthetic result. Compromising the price or the time needed is likely to result in a poorly made denture. Exceptions should be made only on the recommendation of your dentist.

Poorly made dentures may not meet properly, making it difficult to chew. They may not fit well around the borders. There may not be sufficient suction between the gums and dentures to maintain stability during eating or speaking. They may push your lips out too much or not enough. Incorrectly made dentures can make you look older or artificially young. There are hundreds of such variables to consider in designing a long-lasting, quality product.

Dentures that Fit

Inexpensive dentures may not be the best choice for quality fit and comfort. Each plate, upper and lower, has to be meticulously shaped for a custom fit.

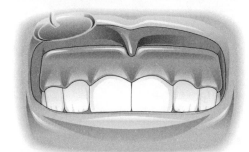

The labial frenum notch must be perfect for the maximum comfort of the denture.

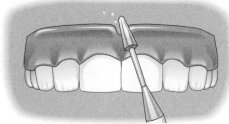

Even with molding techniques, the notch has to be shaped with trimming burs and polishers.

Denture adhesive use is a sticky situation

I've been using denture adhesives for more than five years. Do they damage your gums? What brand or brands would you recommend?

Continued use of any product in the mouth can cause changes in the type and amounts of bacteria. However, denture adhesives don't warrant concern. They have been implicated in allergic reactions, and some researchers suggest they cause bone beneath a denture to resorb faster, but there is little evidence to support either claim.

That Extra Something

Wafer inserts to make dentures fit more snugly should be prescribed by your dentist. Paste adhesives that are soluble are usually the best choice. Be aware of "dentures fit-like-gloves" kits.

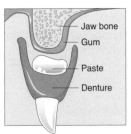

Denture pastes are a soluble adhesive for the bonding of denture to gum.

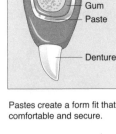

Pastes create a form fit that is comfortable and secure.

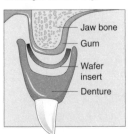

Wafer inserts are also soluble and help to secure a loose fit.

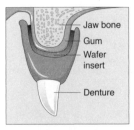

Wafers are safer than do-it-yourself denture kits. Consult your dentist before choosing a denture adhesive.

Denture adhesives are used by about 20 percent of the nation's estimated 45 million denture wearers. Americans spent $148 million on adhesives last year. Since there are many products to choose from, the American Dental Association Seal of Approval is recommended to ensure a quality product.

Adhesives seal the denture to the gum and bone. The material swells 50 to 150 percent, filling the voids and stabilizing the denture.

A loose denture that requires adhesives may need to be remade. Many well-made dentures stay in place without adhesives, relying on a natural suction created by the denture and gums.

After several years the underlying bone may deteriorate, and the denture may need to be relined or replaced.

A dentist relines a denture by filling voids (where it no longer makes contact with the gum) with an acrylic plastic. Your dentures should be relined or adjusted at least every five years.

Getting a grip on an irksome denture fit

My father is frustrated with his third set of dentures. Still, after several years, he complains that they don't fit well and he can't use them. What can be done?

Recent studies estimate that 25 percent of denture wearers have severe problems with their dentures. Complaints range from looseness and pain to difficulties in eating and speaking.

Three variables are most often cited in research that analyzes the reasons for dissatisfied denture wearers. How well the denture is made, the functional limitations of dentures and a patient's expectations head the complaint lists. Your father's frustration is likely described by the latter two categories. Since your father has had three sets of dentures made, the quality has been addressed by three competent dentists. If one was not a prosthodontist, a specialist who concentrates in this area, then a fourth set may be worth making. At best, dentures can only accomplish one-third the function and comfort of your natural teeth. How well they function is largely determined by the amount and contour of the bone in your jaws since they support the dentures. The best-made denture on little or no ridge of bone can be frustrating for any person.

In such cases, dental implants or fixtures that adhere to bone may help stabilize and hold dentures in place. The procedure is easy and safe and may provide a new approach to an old problem of missing teeth.

Expectations of people wearing dentures is another factor determining how well a denture is accepted. For first-time denture wearers, these expectations of how well their new teeth will function have to be continually realized

Secure Dentures

There are a few reasons why some dentures refuse to fit no matter how well-made. One is that there is little bone structure to adhere to the dentures. Dentures that are loose or cause pain because of bad fit can be secured by anchors or bars and connectors.

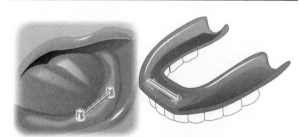

A bar connector is attached to the bone of the patient to anchor the lower dentures.

A bar sleeve is soldered to the framework of the lower dentures.

and reinforced. Try not to let the disappointment of a procedure get in the way of your relationship and trust in your dentist. By letting your dentist know your concerns and frustrations, he or she may be better able to help you adjust to these problems or suggest an alternate procedure or specialist.

Dentures are suspect in appearance of sores

*Ever since wearing my new dentures, I've developed sores
at the corners of my mouth. They haven't healed in several weeks,
and I'm worried. How could they have started and what can
I do to get rid of them?*

Sores Caused by Dentures

The vertical dimension of the dentures sometimes causes sores in the corner of the mouth.

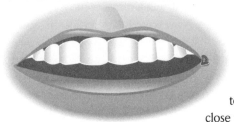

Your sores may be directly linked to your new dentures, especially if they appeared at or near the time you started wearing them. In addition to the functions of chewing, speaking and appearance, dentures also define how your teeth contact each other when you close your mouth. Dentists describe this as the vertical dimension.

If the dentures have a *closed vertical dimension,* closing more than normal, the corners of your lips fold in as you close. Saliva will keep an otherwise dry area moist. Eventually, sores form and will usually remain unless the position of the teeth on the dentures is changed.

The condition, called angular cheilitis or perleche, may get worse. Often, microorganisms such as staph or strep, or fungal growths can form in these moist areas. Ongoing sores begin to form crust at the edges. Patients may experience a burning sensation.

Other factors may cause these sores. Riboflavin and iron deficiency anemia can cause angular cheilitis as well as trauma or injury to the lips.

Finding the cause or causes of the sores is the only permanent course of treatment. Correction of the biting planes of your dentures, vitamin supplements or antibiotic and anti-fungal ointments can then be used to treat the sores.

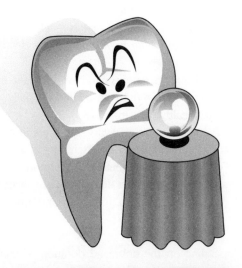

Chapter 17

"Everything Else"

Radiation advantages are weighed against harm

*My mother is currently undergoing radiation treatment in the head
and neck area. Recently she has had more cavities and complains
that her mouth is always dry. Is it related to the radiation,
and what can we do to prevent further dental problems?*

Radiation treatments can have dramatic effects on teeth and surrounding structures of the mouth. In addition to killing cancerous cells, radiation also damages healthy structures.

Blood vessels and salivary glands are most prone to destruction by ongoing treatments. Without blood vessels, important pathways for carrying nutrients to the bone, tissues and teeth are compromised. These structures then become weakened. Likewise, the destruction of salivary glands decreases and eventually stops the flow of saliva, important in bathing and protecting the surfaces of tissues and teeth.

Osteoradionecrosis describes the weakened condition of the jawbone. Depending on the dose and duration of radiation treatment, this bone will continue to weaken. Dry mouth, or *zerostomia*, is the result of damaged salivary glands. Saliva is important because it contains antibodies and cleans a harmful decay-causing bacteria. When glands producing saliva are destroyed, tooth decay can easily form and spread. The outer surfaces of teeth by the gumline are most prone to this decay.

Fluoride supplements placed on the teeth and artificial salivas can help prevent the increase in tooth decay. But only by limiting the radiation dose can the effects on bone and tissues be controlled. However, that must be weighed against the rate of cancer growth. The degree of oral problems is variable with each person. Therefore, continued regular visits to your dentist to monitor changes is recommended.

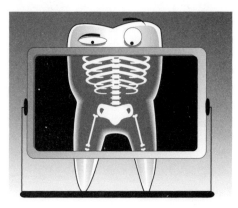

Multiple x-rays ease the detection of problems

Our ten-year-old grandson has had several dental x-rays taken.
What do they show?

Depending on your age, your dentist will select one of five types of x-rays, each valuable in detecting certain problems. Your dentist may take more than one type of x-ray of an area to accurately identify an infection or abnormality.

X-rays are useful in showing the relationship of infection to the teeth, how teeth and surrounding structures relate to each other and how teeth relate to the jaw bones which hold them.

The most common x-ray is the bitewing. It shows the visible areas of teeth in both jaws and parts of their roots. Usually four bitewing x-rays are taken to detect cavities between teeth. Periapical x-rays (taken with an x-ray holder) are taken to view roots and are useful in detecting infection. An occlusal x-ray is a larger film placed between the biting surfaces of all teeth. This film helps your dentist determine if there is adequate space for underlying adult teeth.

Special machines are needed for taking other x-rays that show the relationship of teeth to the jaws and skull. A panoramic x-ray is commonly used by orthodontists and oral surgeons since it shows the lower and base of the skull. A cephalometric x-ray shows the skull. It's used by specialists for treating bone fractures and for other surgical procedures.

Each x-ray provides a unique view which, when combined with other information, gives your dentist a complete picture.

Eliminating anxiety removes gag response

I have a tendency to gag when my dentist takes molds of my teeth
with that gelatin-like material. Can my dentist do anything
to make the process easier?

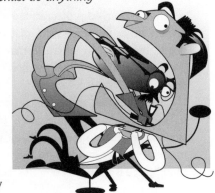

Many people suffer from what's known as a "gag reflex." Involuntary choking, coughing or gagging are common with this reflex (caused by stimulation or a tickling sensation of the palate, tongue and cheek) which often makes routine dental procedures difficult.

If gagging occurs only when your dentist takes molds, the cause can probably be attributed to alginate, or the gelatin-like material, which tickles the soft palate near the throat. Should the reflex occur at other times, the cause may be tactile stimulation of other areas of the mouth or anxiety.

Share your concerns with your dentist. Talking out the steps in a procedure can ease fears. The tickling sensation can be relieved through anesthetics such as topical gels or sprays that numb. Specialized techniques in taking impressions can be used on those who still are unable to control the reflex. Sitting upright and tilting your head forward during the impression can reduce the sensation that the material is creeping down your throat.

Custom mouthguard offers the best protection

Our son plays on a local football team, and we'd like to know what the best mouthguard is to protect his teeth.

There are three types of mouthguards: 1) stock-type, 2) mouth-formed, and 3) custom-made. I would recommend seeing your dentist for a custom-made guard, which most dentists feel provides the best protection.

The stock-type, usually found at sporting goods stores, consists of a rubber or plastic shell in the form of a dental arch. It does not adapt to the teeth and therefore fits loosely. Because it is held by biting pressure, breathing is often restricted.

Mouth-formed protectors are made of a softer material and thus can adapt somewhat to the teeth. The material, however, eventually breaks down and causes the guard to loosen. It may also be bulky, depending upon the brand. Some of the newer mouth-formed protectors would make an adequate second choice when cost is a factor.

Custom-made mouthguards meet all standards of safety and are the only type recommended by the dental profession. Your dentist will take an impression of the teeth to make a plaster model. The plastic guard is made from this model, and later fitted to the teeth. Although more expensive, a custom-made mouthpiece is the most comfortable and can be worn for longer periods of time.

Gaps between teeth aggravate shifting

I'm a 56-year-old woman. During middle age, do teeth move?
My dentist recently took some x-rays, and he noticed a shifting of my teeth.
Is that due to my age and what causes it?

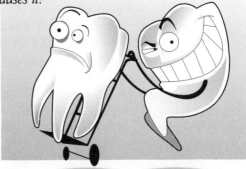

Teeth move throughout your life. They continue to slowly drift forward even after the adult teeth are in place. If you've lost an adult tooth or have an abnormal space between certain teeth, the adjacent teeth may begin to shift toward that empty space.

For example, if you've lost a lower molar tooth, teeth on either side of the space will drift together and may also rotate. A tooth above the space in your upper jaw can move slightly downward towards the space.

These movements will cause changes in the way your teeth meet as you bite. One example of such a change is a premature contact when biting, causing undue tooth stress. Such movements or premature contacts are gradual but may cause chronic jaw pain in later years.

How should such spaces be treated? Restoring the contact relationship between teeth with a fixed or removable appliance is the solution of choice. Such a space should be filled with an artificial tooth. This will maintain contact with surrounding teeth in place of the missing tooth.

In addition, reconstruction should be done in such a way as to evenly distribute the load carried by the surrounding teeth. The sooner this is completed, the more likely the reconstruction will match the position of your original teeth.

All this reader wants is two front teeth

How come certain teeth are naturally absent in people,
not from accidents or decay? Everyone in my family
has normal teeth, but I'm missing my two front teeth.

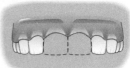

The absence of permanent teeth or *partial anodontia* is common. However, its cause is not clear. Genetics appear to be a principal factor, and yet only ten percent of those affected have any family history of missing teeth.

The teeth most commonly missing are lower second premolar teeth and upper lateral incisors (the teeth next to your two front teeth). Other teeth can be missing as well. Eighty-eight percent of the time, a person is missing only one or two teeth. Seldom are more teeth absent.

Problems often arise when teeth are missing. Functional and aesthetic problems are common, as other teeth are usually out of normal position. In addition, abnormal spaces result between teeth.

Because the problem may be detected at an early age, positioning of the teeth can be corrected during normal growth and development. Combining this with restorative procedures, an odd space or tooth shape can be changed to look normal.

Anesthetic injections can be a real pain

I've always hated shots and fear the worst every time I see the dentist. But how come some shots are so painful and others I hardly notice?

Many factors determine how sensitive an injection of anesthetic can be. Among them are location of the injection, amount of infection around the area of concern, the temperature of the anesthetic solution, the rate of injection, your body's metabolic rate and mental anticipation.

If you have one bad experience with an injection, you will often anticipate a similar experience, even if subsequent experiences are without incident. For this reason, it is important to have regular checkups to avoid difficult problems that may complicate the injection. Infections, for example, can neutralize the effect of the anesthetic, making it more difficult for the dentist to numb an area.

Generally, the warmer the anesthetic solution, the less sensitive the injection. Slowly injecting the anesthetic over a couple of minutes is less sensitive than a more rapid injection. Injections into wide, soft tissue spaces surrounding the cheeks and jaws are less sensitive than into tissue thinly stretched over bone, such as the palate and gums near the base of your teeth. Because these factors affect the sensitivity of an injection, your dentist will often try to warn you of sensations you can expect to feel.

Life loses its flavor as taste buds waver

My grandfather says that older people lose their sense of taste over time. He uses that as an excuse when he doesn't eat as much as we'd like him to. Is there any truth to his theory?

About half of your taste buds will not be functioning by age 70. The sense of smell is also affected during the aging process.

Because of these diminished senses, older people may lose their appetite more frequently, and the decrease in food consumption can be a problem. For example, vitamins C and B deficiencies can cause changes in the color and health of oral tissues. Gums may become swollen, ulcers develop and bleeding arise.

Malnutrition also may lower resistance to other infections and affect overall general health.

Many conditions of the body and mouth can contribute to the loss of appetite. Medications with a side effect of decreasing saliva flow can affect chewing and swallowing. An ill-fitting denture may interfere with eating. Other painful dental or gum infections make eating more difficult and likewise may contribute to malnutrition.

Regular visits to the dentist may identify factors that contribute to poor eating habits. By observing changes in the oral tissues, your dentist can identify vitamin deficiencies and refer you to a dietician for any further counseling and treatment.

Tell dentist if you've had beer before visit

My husband sometimes has a beer before going to the dentist. Can this cause problems?

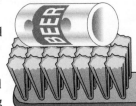

The effects of alcohol can interfere with many dental procedures.

A drink before a dental visit can determine how long an anesthetic will last.

It also can have detrimental effects if antibiotics or pain medications are taken after treatment. Aspirin and other anti-inflammatory drugs can cause severe stomach pain when combined with alcohol.

If your husband is taking any type of anticoagulant, bleeding can be prolonged with alcohol use. Any consumption of alcohol after treatment can affect the outcome of a procedure. For example, tooth-colored materials called composites soften with alcohol exposure. Healing after dental and oral surgery takes longer.

If this drink before the dental visit reflects a deeper habit or even abuse, there are additional concerns. Heavy drinkers have a ten percent greater chance of developing oral cancer. They also suffer more from gum disease and other oral infections.

A heavy drinker is defined as one whose "average daily consumption is one ounce or more of ethanol each day" (that's about two cocktails, beers or glasses of wine.)

It's estimated that 25 percent of dental patients are classified as heavy drinkers.

Your husband should inform your dentist of his drink before the dental visit so that necessary precautions can be taken. A continued drinking habit should be limited or stopped to prevent additional complications and risks.

Lack of saliva hinders the ability to taste

My 90-year-old bedridden mother frequently complains that she cannot taste her food. Her mouth has been dry since she began radiation treatment. Can her dry mouth affect tasting, and what can we do to help?

People who lack salivary function often complain about an inability to taste. Although past research concluded that saliva is necessary for a normal sense of taste, recent findings indicate otherwise. Current studies at the National Institute for Dental Research state: "Some individuals who had complete failure of salivary systems still maintained normal taste."

Your mother's dry mouth is only partially preventing her from enjoying her food. Saliva contains enzymes that break food into smaller units which have a unique taste of their own. When you eat fruitcake, for example, part of your ability to distinguish the flavors of cherries and walnuts comes from tasting the food before it is broken down and part from a taste of the piece that the enzyme breaks apart.

You can help your mother by serving her moistened food or dry food served with liquids to help dissolve the food and make swallowing easier.

You may want to consult your dentist on the use of artificial salivas designed for people with dry mouths.

Oral piercing, the hole story

My daughter is talking about having her tongue pierced.
Who performs this operation and is it safe?

Tongue and lip piercing are the most common forms of body piercing that directly affect the oral cavity. Tongue piercing is rapidly catching up to navel piercing as the most common site. The fad which began several years ago continues in its popularity. The operation can be performed by accredited piercers, but unfortunately many others are inadequately trained. As a result, there can be serious consequences including prolonged bleeding, tissue infections, and infections spreading in the body's blood stream which can be fatal.

After insertion of the oral jewelry, surrounding tissue is always prone to infection and needs to be monitored regularly. Symptoms resulting from the procedure include pain, swelling and redness. Ongoing effects to the surrounding oral cavity include damage to existing restorations and natural teeth, and gum and bone defects that result from the abrasion and trauma of the ornament against the tissue. Because of these adverse effects, most dentists strictly advise against oral piercing.

There are several observations that can help direct you to a safer piercer. First, avoid salons that use a piercing gun as opposed to a needle. Second, the piercing of the tongue should begin from the underside to avoid damage to blood vessels. Third, if the salon or studio doesn't look as clean as your dentist's office, take your tongue to a new location. There are national organizations for hygiene and proof of these should be prominently displayed.

It's a matter of taste when it comes to food.

Every Thanksgiving my brother and I disagree about the taste of our grandmother's cranberry sauce. He says it's bitter; I say it's sweet. Is it possible to have such different tastes?

Yes. People who are unable to taste bitter foods are "taste blind."

Sensitivity to bitter is controlled by heredity, specifically a single gene. If you lack this gene, you'll never taste anything bitter.

Taste is usually broken down into four categories: sweet, sour, salty and bitter – and it differs from our other senses, like sight. The eye sees a mixture of red and yellow as orange, but in the mouth, each taste is recognized.

Some flavorings and condiments, however, have a property called "synergy", where one taste brings out another. Salt, for example, can bring out a certain taste quality in steak.

Taste is often associated with the tongue, but the soft palate and top portion of your throat also have taste buds. That is why taste, as many researchers have found, is still a mystery. Because none of us has the same number or distribution of taste buds, we all probably taste food differently.

Latex gloves fingered in allergic reactions

I read an article about some dental patients having allergic reactions to latex gloves used by the dentist and staff. What kind of reactions occur and what should be done if an allergy is found?

Latex used in dentistry and medicine can be either a natural or synthetic rubber. Although most latex products used in the health care industry are natural, most allergies are caused by processing chemicals used in manufacturing.

Studies estimate that one percent of the general population has a sensitivity to latex. Health care workers have a five-ten percent rate. For almost all patients and health workers, the risk of an allergic reaction is minimal. Latex has proven to be a valuable and safe material unmatched by any other in the delivery of health care. However, the small numbers of allergies are important to note.

Allergies reported are of two types:

• The most common is a delayed reaction known as allergic contact dermatitis. Symptoms include redness, swelling, itching and even cracking of the skin. They occur about two days after exposure.

• The second type is more immediate, usually occurring within seconds or minutes after exposure. Signs include hives, itchy eyes and wheezing. In some instances, a more life-threatening form can occur. Reactions such as difficulty in breathing and lowered blood pressure can result. This immediate reaction is only found with allergies to protein found in natural rubber and does not occur with synthetic rubber products.

People who have either type of allergy should document the condition in all medical and dental records. Additionally, special nonallergic gloves should be worn to avoid continued exposure.

Tooth-decay vaccine still eludes scientists

My family has always had a problem with cavities. I've heard that work is being done to develop a vaccine for tooth decay. Will this be available soon?

Researchers have been working for 20 years on a tooth-decay vaccine, but significant problems stand in the way.

The principle of a vaccine is to first identify the bacteria or virus that causes the infection. The body then is exposed to a form of the bacteria that will not cause the infection but will stimulate the body's immune response. The body then will be prepared to fight off the infection the next time it is exposed to that bacteria.

THE TOOTH DECAY PILL TAKE ONE AND NEVER CALL THE DENTIST AGAIN

The problem with the bacteria which cause tooth decay is that they quickly change to disguise themselves from attack.

In a study at Emory University, student volunteers took capsules of cavity-causing bacteria. Over three months, the immune response worked to clear more than 90 percent of the same bacteria from the mouths of most of the subjects. Later, however, new strains went unrecognized by the subjects' immune systems.

A study at the Harvard University-affiliated Forsyth Dental Center has concentrated on infants near the age of one. Cavity-causing bacteria appear only when teeth first begin to erupt in the mouth. Researchers are trying to find a vaccine that will keep these bacteria from ever developing.

It may seem a distant dream, but studies like these could change dentistry dramatically. You may eventually take a pill to fight cavities.

Saliva change leaves elders disease prone

Does your saliva change as you get older?
At the age of 60 my mouth seems drier,
and I'm beginning to get some cavities.
I'm not taking any medications and otherwise seem healthy.

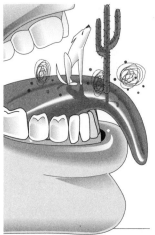

Recent studies have found that your saliva changes with age. Certain changes in the amount and components of saliva have long been associated with medications and disease. Diabetes and salivary gland disorders as well as medications for such problems as hypertension are examples of problems that can directly affect salivary flow. However, there are differences in the components of saliva that change with age even in people who have no illnesses or are taking no medications.

Researchers have found that in the saliva of people over the age of 65 there is much less mucin, a lubricating component of saliva that protects teeth and gums. Mucin also helps to prevent bacterial growth and thus prevents tooth decay and disease. Because of this lack of mucin, seniors may be more prone to cavities and gum problems.

Stimulating the glands by chewing sugarless gum, rinsing with fluoride mouth rinses or brushing with fluoride toothpaste can help to prevent such decay.

The picture of x-ray safety

Are dental x-rays safe?
What is being done to limit radiation exposure?

Yes, x-rays are safe. The dose for a set of four bitewing radiographs is roughly equivalent to the radiation dose received during an airline flight at 39,000 feet for seven hours. Because radiation is cumulative in its effect, the dosage during one's life should be considered against oral health risk factors and prevalence of dental decay.

The concept of ALARA, As Low As Reasonably Achievable has been instituted in current guidelines. In 2005, newer guidelines from the American Dental Association adhere to a conservative approach to x-rays, taking into account the dental health and cavity prevalence for each individual. Among the organizations that advise the use of x-rays in the dental office are the U.S. Food and Drug Administration, the National Council on Radiation Protection and Measurements and the American Academy of Oral and Maxillofacial Radiology. The emphasis continues to be placed on minimizing radiation exposure without compromising the diagnostic ability of your dentist.

Factors that limit radiation exposure include film speed, design of the x-ray machine and newer digital technology that utilizes a sensor instead of film. Advances in technology combined with decreasing the frequency of films taken in accordance with initial need, make dental x-rays more safe for patients.

"Wood I lie?" George's teeth made of ivory

What kind of teeth did George Washington have?
Every time his birthday rolls around, I get curious,
especially since I've read that they were not made of wood.

The question from the original game Trivial Pursuit asks, "What were George Washington's false teeth made of?" The answer-"Wood", when in fact there is not a splinter of wood showing on the President's false teeth. How did history get it wrong on what may be the most renowned false teeth in America. And, if not wood, what were they made of?

The teeth are made of ivory, the jaw portion gold, and they are held together by two stainless steel springs. Some wood dowels were used to hold the teeth in place, but wood was, by no means, the material that identified the President's dentures. The maker was Dr. John Greenwood who was Washington's dentist for many years. In 1789 he extracted the President's last tooth and provided a new set of dentures. In all, there were four sets of false teeth made. Materials used for the teeth on these dentures varied from hippopotamus and elephant tusk to human teeth. Most of the work was credited to Dr. Greenwood although debate continues about the maker of one lead set reported to be used for presidential portrait work.

Chapter 17: "Everything Else"

Just how did the story of Washington's teeth get out of alignment? During the period, it was common for professionals to write papers on the treatment they provided. One such paper had a section which stated, " During Washington's time, some poor people had to wear teeth of wood." Twenty years later another dentist, who felt this section was worth repeating, changed a word or two to read " Even Washington, in his time, wore teeth of wood." From there the rumor spread and continues to be the adhesive that sticks to this denture story today.

History continues to go awry when Paul Revere's name gets attached as the maker of the teeth. Although the silversmith practiced dentistry for several years after the economic downturn following the French and Indian War, Washington was not one of his patients.

If you've ever examined any of Washington's many portraits, you may find some odd expressions on his face. A dentist may be able to describe these looks better than any of the original painters. The portrait hanging in the Philadelphia Academy of Fine Arts, for example, shows Washington with a bulge on the side of his face. This was due to a tooth abcess. To make other portraits look normal, the President's lips were padded with cotton to restore the natural lines of his lips. The president had so many dental problems that even his hair-trigger temper was thought to be related to his on-going problems with his teeth.